Keith L. Belvin

12 Steps to Recovering from A Toxic Relationship

by

Keith K. L. Belvin, MHSC, MS Ed

Bravin Publishing USA, Delaware / New York

12 Steps to Recovering from A Toxic Relationship

Keith L. Belvin

Dedication

I want to dedicate this book to my lovely wife, Tiffany, who helps remind me daily what a solid positive relationship looks and feels like. Your Love and Support keep me grounded. To all my children, Johnathan, Kierra, Anthony, Elijah, Courtney, Justin, and Kayelle, I have had positive and negative times with all of you. I pray the Lord will continue to cover and bless you in whatever direction life takes all of you. Know that I am here whenever you need me. Your Dad Loves You! To my late mother, Katrina Belvin, and my late Grandmother, Christina Watkins, may you both continue to Rest in Peace.

You both played a significant role in shaping me into the man I've become. In your time here on earth, you have been through your share of toxic relationships with family, friends, and partners over your lifetime. Thank you for fighting through all the negatives to pour into this boy who grew into an optimistic man. I also dedicate this book to every person who has removed themselves from a relationship that was hurting them but is now on the pathway to healing. To my Heavenly Father, thank you for allowing me to use my writing talents to reach other brothers and sisters who need assistance. Thank You, Father, for your Grace. This book will change lives for the better. Keith K. L. Belvin, MHSC, MS Ed. "A Happily Divorced and Happily Remarried" Crisis Specialist and Human Service Counselor.

12 Steps to Recovering from A Toxic Relationship

Publication Page

Published by

Bravin Publishing

Copyright © 2023 Keith K. L. Belvin, MHSC, MS Ed.

All rights reserved, including the right of reproduction in whole or part in any form. No part of this book may be used or reproduced in any manner whatsoever without permission except in the case of brief quotations embodied in critical articles and reviews.

ISBN:
978-1-7355290-9-7

Library of Congress Control Number: 2023912433

Printed in the United States of America

Keith L. Belvin

Table of Contents

Acknowledgments 12
Foreword 13
Self-Assessment Quiz: Identifying Toxic Patterns 27
Introduction 30
Step 1: Accept Your Current Mental and Emotional Positioning with Your Life 33
    Allow yourself to feel your emotions. 33
    Take care of your physical health. 34
    Practice self-compassion. 35
    Seek support from others. 35
    Set boundaries. 36
    Focus on the present. 38
    Cultivate gratitude. 39
    Let go of guilt or shame: 40
    Create a new routine: 41
    Celebrate your progress. 42
Step 2: Pay Close Attention To How You Got To This Point 44
    Reflect on your past. 44
    Identify your triggers. 45
    Assess your boundaries. 47
    Review your communication style. 48
    Explore your values. 49
    Evaluate your self-esteem. 50

12 Steps to Recovering from A Toxic Relationship

Analyze your support system. 51

Reflect on your decision-making process. 52

Assess your coping mechanisms: 54

Set goals for the future: 55

Step 3: Don't Blame Yourself For Your Part In The Toxic Relationship 58

Acknowledge that relationships involve two people. ... 58

Practice self-compassion, ... 60

Reflect on your role in the relationship. 62

Accept that you cannot control the other person. 63

Seek feedback from trusted friends and family. 65

Focus on your personal growth. 67

Let go of guilt and shame. 69

Avoid self-blame and negative self-talk. 70

Take responsibility for your part, but don't take on all the blame. 72

Move forward with a positive attitude: 74

Step 4: Offer Yourself Patience and Grace 77

Recognize that healing takes time. 77

Practice self-care. 79

Set boundaries for yourself and others. 80

Journal your feelings. 82

Seek support. 83

Reach out to friends, family, or a therapist during this challenging time. 85

Forgive yourself. 86

Let go of any shame or guilt. 88

Practice self-compassion. 89

Engage in positive activities. 91

Step 5. Face Your Pain, Don't Be Scare To Accept Your Discomfort 94

Acknowledge your pain. 94

Be kind to yourself. 96

Seek support, ... 98

Practice self-care. 100

Identify your triggers. 101

Let yourself grieve. 103

Forgive yourself. 105

Engage in positive activities. 106

Be patient. 108

Accept discomfort: 110

Step 6: Getting Closure Is On You, Not The Person Who Hurt You. 113

Acknowledge your feelings. 113

Recognize that closure comes from within. 117

Reframe the situation. 118

Forgive yourself. 120

Create closure rituals: 122

Focus on the present. 124

Practice self-care. 125

Seek professional help if needed.................................. 127
Celebrate your progress. 129
***Closure Rituals: ***... 131
Step 7: How To Keep Supportive People Around You
After Getting Out Of Toxic Relationship 132
   Identify your support system: 132
   Reach out to them. 134
   Be honest about your needs. 136
   Make time for them. 137
   Practice self-care. 139
   Seek out therapy. 140
   Join a support group. 142
   Set boundaries. 144
   Express gratitude. 146
   Be open to new relationships. 147
Step 8: How to Redefine Personal Happiness................. 150
   Identify and prioritize your values: 150
   Practice self-care. 152
   Explore new hobbies or interests. 154
   Set achievable goals for yourself. 156
   Surround yourself with positive and supportive people.
   157
   Practice gratitude. 159
   Practice forgiveness: 161

Reconnect with old friends or family members. 163
Seek professional counseling or therapy 164
Take time to reflect. 166
Step 9: Stay Grounded In Their Current Position 169
Practice self-care: 169
Build a support network. 171
Set boundaries. 173
Cultivate a positive mindset. 174
Find healthy coping methods. 176
Practice forgiveness. 177
Learn from the experience. 179
Find ways to stay connected to your passions. 180
Create a vision for your future. 182
Celebrate your progress: 184
****S.M.A.R.T. Goals**** 186
Step 10: How a Person Can Care For Themselves, Physically, Mentally, Emotionally, and Spiritually. 188
Practice self-compassion: 188
Take care of your physical health. 190
Find healthy ways to manage stress. 192
Seek professional support. 193
Connect with supportive people. 195
Set boundaries. 197
Pursue your passions. 198
Practice mindfulness. 200

12 Steps to Recovering from A Toxic Relationship

    Get creative. 201

    Connect with your spiritual side. 203

Step 11: Practice Self-Kindness. "Speak Life into Yourself." 206

    Practice self-compassion. 206

    Take time for yourself. 208

    Set healthy boundaries. 209

    Engage in positive self-talk. 211

    Cultivate a positive mindset: 212

    Practice forgiveness. 214

    Engage in activities that promote relaxation. 215

    Celebrate your accomplishments. 217

    Practice self-care. 218

    Surround yourself with positive people. 219

"Speak Life Into Yourself" Quotes: 223

Step 12: Don't Check In On Your Ex Once Out Of Your Negative Situation 224

    Delete their contact information and unfollow them on social media. 224

    Replace the urge to check in with a different activity, such as exercise or a hobby. 226

    Reach out to supportive friends or family members for distraction and encouragement. 228

    Journal about feelings of loneliness or sadness instead of acting on the urge to check in. 229

Remind yourself of the reasons why the relationship was toxic and why it is vital to move on. 231

Seek professional help or counseling to process difficult emotions and thoughts. 232

Create a daily self-care routine that includes activities that bring you joy and fulfillment. 233

Use positive affirmations or mantras to shift your mindset and focus on self-improvement. 235

Set healthy boundaries with your ex and communicate clearly about your needs and expectations. 237

Focus on personal growth and development, such as taking a class or pursuing a new career opportunity... 238

"Don't Check On Your Ex Quotes". 241

Additional Resources - I 242

Additional Resources - II. 245

Who Is Keith K. L. Belvin, MHSC, MS Ed.? 248

12 Steps to Recovering from A Toxic Relationship

Keith L. Belvin

Acknowledgments

My brother from another mother, Brian Groves, thank you for all the kicks with kindness you have given me over the years as a mentor and friend.

To Glenn P. Brooks Jr. and Sheri Brooks, for your role as my business coaches and friends, Glenn, your guidance has helped me understand my gifts and how to use them to help others.

To Tar'kesa Colvin, you have, in your way, help reshaped my professional and literary life with your teaching and your service to the Lord. Thank you.

To the MMC, I want to thank you in the business community for the love and support you have shown me.

To Justin Sensesi and your family, thank you for what you have allowed me to do for you and the service provided to the Hickory Ridge Church family in the name of the Lord.

To Jennifer J on Tik Tok, thank you for gifting me the idea of writing this book and explaining to me the potential of its power of helping those hurting after getting out of a bad situation.

12 Steps to Recovering from A Toxic Relationship

Foreword

Have you ever been in a toxic relationship that left you feeling drained, broken, and unworthy? Have you struggled to move on and find healing after leaving that relationship behind? If so, you're not alone.

As someone who has experienced multiple toxic relationships, I know firsthand how challenging it can be to recover and start anew. But I also know it's possible to heal and find the love and happiness you deserve. That's why I'm excited to introduce you to a remarkable book near and dear to my heart, "12 Steps to Recovering from a Toxic Relationship."

Trust me when I say this is the book you've been searching for. Suppose you're longing to heal from the wounds of a toxic relationship and move forward with newfound confidence. In that case, look no further. "12 Steps to Recovering from a Toxic Relationship" is the game-changer you need. Its pages are filled with practical wisdom, heartfelt guidance, and real-life stories that will resonate with you deeply.

Let me start by being real with you. There was a time when I carried a heavy burden of shame and embarrassment because of my multiple marriages. It felt like a scarlet letter, a glaring sign of failure that I wore on my sleeve. I constantly worried about being judged by others, fearing their whispers and sideways glances.

Keith L. Belvin

Even in my current marriage, it took me years to shake off the nagging feeling that something was inherently wrong with me. I questioned why I seemed to attract the wrong partners and why my marriages always seemed to crumble. It was a painful and confusing journey, filled with self-doubt and moments of deep reflection.

But here's the truth that I finally discovered: I wasn't the problem. It wasn't some inherent flaw in my character that doomed my relationships. No, the root of the issue lay within my inner brokenness, the wounds that had never fully healed. It was this unhealed pain that unconsciously attracted toxic relationships into my life.

Realizing this was a pivotal moment. It shifted my perspective and showed me I wasn't destined for doomed relationships. I wasn't unworthy of love or destined to repeat the same patterns. I had the power to break free from the cycle and rewrite my story. But let me tell you, it wasn't an easy path. It required me to dig deep into my past and confront the traumas that had shaped me. I had to face the pain head-on, acknowledging the wounds that had been silently festering. Through this journey of healing, I began to see my worthiness. I realized I deserved to be in a loving relationship that nurtured and uplifted me.

As I sit down to write this foreword, I can't help but reflect on my journey and the experiences that have brought me to this moment. So, let me introduce myself - I'm Yolanda Marie Tate, a retired United States Army Command Sergeant Major with over 29 years of

12 Steps to Recovering from A Toxic Relationship

dedicated service under my belt. But my career journey doesn't end there. I'm also an IT Professional, a Wellness Consultant, and a Coach who passionately advocates for holistic well-being. At the very essence of who I am, I have a deep passion for empowering others to invest in their wellness. I believe in the power of embracing our whole selves physically, spiritually, mentally, and emotionally. But let me tell you, my journey toward holistic well-being hasn't always been a smooth ride. Life has thrown its fair share of challenges my way, and I've had to face some tough battles head-on. And you know what? Some of the most brutal battles I've encountered have been within the realm of my relationships. Those experiences have left their marks, scars that are invisible to the world but have significantly shaped me into the resilient person I am today. I proudly admit that I'm a work in progress, fully aware that personal growth is a continuous daily journey.

Toxic relationships can hit anyone, coming in all shapes and sizes. Emotional abuse, physical abuse, financial abuse, even sexual abuse – the impact can be devastating. They leave you feeling depleted, shattered, and questioning your worth. But here's the kicker: sometimes, we don't even realize we're trapped in a toxic relationship. We wear these blinders, dismissing the warning signs, especially when in love or desperately seeking companionship. Yet, as time passes, those signs become harder to brush aside. The key lies in spotting them early on and taking action. And here's the real kicker: that action begins with YOU, not the other person. It's about working on yourself, prioritizing your well-being, and choosing a healthier path.

In my journey, I had to face the truth and take responsibility for my actions. It was a tough pill to swallow, but I realized that toxic relationships often arise from both parties carrying unresolved wounds and childhood traumas. It meant confronting the pain of not knowing my father and lacking strong father figures in my life. Growing up in Philly, I didn't witness many loving, two-parent relationships. Like me, most of my friends were navigating life without a father in the home or with a father who was physically present but emotionally absent. It was a common thread that ran through our experiences.

Growing up without a father profoundly impacted me, leaving a lingering sense of longing and insecurity. It influenced my relationship choices, and I always attracted the wrong partners. At one point, I even adopted the mindset of being the "I don't need a man... I can handle everything on my own" kind of woman. But deep down, I knew that to break free from these negative patterns, and I had to embark on a journey of self-reflection and inner healing. I recognized that to overcome my past wounds, I had to put in the work and confront my traumas head-on.

Let me tell you, it was far from an easy journey. In fact, it was one of the most challenging things I've ever done. I had to dig deep and embark on a soul-searching mission, facing some painful truths about myself along the way. It meant acknowledging my

12 Steps to Recovering from A Toxic Relationship

brokenness and accepting my role in attracting toxic relationships. Believe me, it was a humbling experience, but it was also incredibly liberating. I rolled up my sleeves and sought therapy and support, which became essential in my journey. Let me be honest with you – this transformation didn't happen overnight. It was and still is a gradual process of self-discovery and growth. It required a deep well of self-compassion, patience, and unwavering perseverance. There were setbacks and moments of doubt, but I held onto the belief that this journey was worth every ounce of effort, and it indeed is.

So, let's go on a trip down memory lane, back to my high school days when my first marriage began taking shape. We were just a couple of young, starry-eyed teenagers with big dreams for the future. Little did I know that toxic behaviors were silently brewing beneath the surface of our seemingly perfect romance? In hindsight, I can now spot the red flags I so naively ignored. I brushed them aside, convincing myself that I was deeply in love and that things would eventually change for the better. But boy, was I wrong. Before long, the verbal and physical abuse began, and I found myself trapped in a cycle of making excuses for his behavior. I kept holding onto the belief that love could conquer all, even when it meant sacrificing my well-being.

Deep down, I had this gut feeling that tying the knot at such a young age was a big mistake. My mom, bless her heart, did everything she could to dissuade me, but I stubbornly went against all advice and went through with it anyway. At that time, I was already serving on Active Duty, stationed at my first duty assignment, while he was an Army Reservist with his own set of obligations.

Little did I know that things would take a sharp nosedive once we said those vows. The person I thought I knew so well seemed to morph into someone possessive and downright abusive. Suspicion oozed from him like poison, especially concerning my friends and male co-workers. And let me tell you, the accusations that would fly if I ever dared to come home later than expected were beyond maddening. The irony was that I was going about my life as any dedicated soldier would, with not a shred of wrongdoing in sight.

The final straw came crashing down on a Friday night. A girlfriend of mine invited me to a much-needed Girls' Night Out. My first husband and I discussed this week prior, and he seemed okay. Little did I know the atmosphere would shift dramatically that evening.

As I stood in front of the mirror, getting ready for the night ahead, I heard the sound of stumbling footsteps approaching the bedroom. My heart skipped a beat as I turned to see him standing there, his breath heavy with the scent of alcohol. His eyes met mine, and in a tone laced with jealousy and anger, he uttered those chilling words, "You're looking too good to go out."

At that moment, a wave of fear washed over me. I knew all too well what would follow. His simmering anger would erupt into a storm of emotional turmoil and possibly physical violence. It was a sinking feeling, a heaviness that settled deep within my chest.

It started as a heated argument, escalating into physical abuse I never thought I would endure. I remember being forcefully pushed against the wall, feeling the air leave my lungs as his hands wrapped around my throat. In that terrifying moment, something snapped within me, and an instinctive surge of strength surged through my body. I managed to muster the courage to knee him where it hurt, giving me the precious seconds, I needed to escape.

Without a second thought, I sprinted out of our apartment, tears streaming down my face, panic gripping my heart. Desperation carried me towards the safe haven of my friend's house, just a couple of blocks away. As I reached her driveway, the sound of a speeding car echoed behind me, sending chills down my spine. Fear and sheer terror consumed me, and I screamed for help, hoping that someone would intervene. Suddenly, my world turned upside down as I felt a brutal body slam, my vision blurred, and darkness began to seep in.

Thankfully, my friend and her husband rushed outside, sensing the urgency in my screams. In that moment of chaos, my friend ran to my side, offering her comforting presence like a lifeline. As she provided solace and support, her husband stepped forward to confront my first ex-husband, effectively restraining him. The commotion caused a gathering of their neighbors, and they swiftly dialed emergency services, ensuring that justice would be served.

That incident marked the turning point when I vowed never to allow him to lay his hands on me again. He was arrested that night, but I chose not to press charges. However, my Army chain of command and comrades provided unwavering support, ensuring my safety and assisting me in getting him a one-way ticket back to Philly, where he belonged.

It took two long years for him to finally sign the divorce papers, freeing me from the shackles of a toxic marriage that had tarnished my spirit. Those years were not without their struggles, but with the love and support of those around me, I slowly pieced my life back together.

Sharing this raw and personal experience with you is not easy, but it is worth it if it can provide solace or strength to even one person facing a similar situation. No one deserves to endure abuse, and no one should ever feel trapped in a toxic relationship.

Now, let's buckle up for the wild ride that was my second marriage. Although it may not have reached the toxicity levels of my first, it had its own hurdles to overcome. You see, my husband battled alcoholism, and that struggle cast a shadow over our relationship. But let me be crystal clear: despite his demons, he has always been a good person at heart. His words never failed to touch me deeply, as he would lovingly call me his beautiful black queen. Those precious words held a special place in my heart, reminding me of the love that did exist amidst the chaos.

But here's the thing: I was still dealing with the lingering brokenness from my first marriage and childhood without a father. It was like carrying around a heavy backpack filled with unresolved emotions. On top of that, my military career demanded much of my focus, and I had my precious son to take care of as well. If you're curious, my son isn't from my first husband - that's a whole different story that could fill its own book.

During this time, I found myself lacking the mindset, patience, strength, and time to confront my brokenness while simultaneously dealing with my husband's struggles. It felt like an overwhelming juggling act, and I realized I needed to make a tough decision. I chose to end the marriage, despite his reluctance to do so. We tried counseling, hoping it would save us, but deep down, I had become emotionally and mentally detached from the marriage.

As we began the divorce process, a glimmer of hope emerged amidst the heartache. During this time, I embarked on a journey of healing from my brokenness. I realized that I needed to focus on myself from a surface level and a more holistic perspective. It was time to dig deep, confront my past traumas, and embrace the path of self-discovery.

I delved into different healing modalities, exploring therapy and self-help books and connecting with supportive communities. The process wasn't easy, and there were moments when I questioned if I had made the right decision. But as I immersed myself in this transformative journey, I gradually regained my sense of self and found a newfound strength.

Looking back, I recognize that my second marriage served as a catalyst for my personal growth. It was pivotal when I acknowledged that I deserved more than simply surviving in relationships. I deserved to thrive, be loved unconditionally, and embrace my worth. The challenges I faced in that marriage pushed me to look hard at myself and prioritize my healing.

Alright, let's fast forward to the present moment. I'm in my third marriage, and we're about to celebrate a remarkable 18 years together. Before you start envisioning a picture-perfect fairytale, let me assure you that our relationship is anything but flawless. No relationship is. Like any other couple, we've had our fair share of ups and downs. But this time is different because we're both deeply committed to the ongoing journey of personal growth, healing, and improving our communication skills.

Let me tell you, and it's no walk in the park. We've had to confront our imperfections, face our deepest insecurities, and work through the challenges of sharing a life together. But through it all, we've learned that commitment isn't just about saying "I do" and coasting through the years. It's about showing up, day in and day out, ready to put in the effort to make our relationship thrive.

12 Steps to Recovering from A Toxic Relationship

One of the areas we've mainly focused on is communication. We've realized that open, honest, and respectful communication is the lifeblood of any healthy relationship. We're still learning to listen attentively, express our needs and concerns, and seek understanding before jumping to conclusions. It's an ongoing process that we continue to grow in every day.

Again, I'm so excited about this book, "12 Steps to Recovering from a Toxic Relationship." It's not just another self-help guide; it's a comprehensive roadmap designed to help you heal, grow, and move forward. This book is packed with practical steps and powerful tools to guide your recovery journey.

One of the things that sets this book apart is its holistic approach. It recognizes that healing goes beyond just the mind or body – it also encompasses the spirit. Each chapter addresses different aspects of your well-being, providing you with a well-rounded framework for transformation. This book covers everything from understanding the signs of toxicity to learning how to set healthy boundaries. And what makes this book unique is that it is written from the depths of personal experience. My friend, Keith L. Belvin, understands the grueling challenges of recovering from a toxic relationship and has compiled his knowledge and experience into this book to help others. His personal and professional credentials make him the perfect person to write this book.

Let me introduce you to Keith, someone who has significantly impacted my life since we crossed paths nearly three years ago. Believe it or not, our connection started on a social media platform called Clubhouse, where we found ourselves drawn to a morning room called Lessons Learned in Business and Ministry. Coach Glenn P Brooks Jr. led this great space. Glenn and his wife, Sheri, have built a vibrant business community called the MMC Business Builder Academy and a supportive relationship community called Marriages and Parenting Successfully (M.A.P.S).

Keith and I decided to join the MMC Business Academy and ended up in the same cohort. During this time, I truly got to know Keith on a deeper level. He wasn't just an entrepreneur with a wealth of knowledge but also an exceptional man, a loving husband, and a dedicated father. What struck me the most was his unwavering commitment to personal growth and his journey to healing from toxic relationships. Keith's passion for helping others navigate their healing journeys, including myself, was truly inspiring.

Last year, Keith and I had the privilege of attending Coach Glenn's "Bootstrapping Your Way to Success Redefined Conference." This event allowed us to share more of our personal stories and engage in meaningful discussions about the profound effects of toxic relationships. It was a spiritual experience filled with transparent and vulnerable moments where we laughed, cried, and expressed our gratitude to God for allowing us to see how our experiences could serve as a source of help and support for others.

12 Steps to Recovering from A Toxic Relationship

What sets Keith apart is his clinical expertise, vast knowledge, and personal experiences. He has walked the path of healing, carrying the scars of toxic relationships and transforming them into valuable lessons that empower others. As someone who has overcome the challenges of toxic relationships firsthand, Keith intimately understands the pain, confusion, and self-doubt that can arise from such experiences. He knows what it takes to heal and rebuild a life filled with love, joy, and healthy connections.

Through his journey, Keith has become a beacon of hope for those seeking guidance and support. His warm, compassionate, and straightforward approach creates a safe space where individuals feel understood and supported as they navigate their healing process. With his unique combination of personal experience and professional expertise, Keith brings a wealth of knowledge to help others overcome the lasting impact of toxic relationships and reclaim their lives.

I am genuinely thrilled that Keith has chosen to share his wisdom and insights through this book. His relatable and down-to-earth writing style will make you feel like you're engaged in a heartfelt conversation with a trusted friend. Whether you're just beginning your healing journey or have been on it for a while, Keith's words will resonate deeply, providing you with the guidance, tools, and actionable steps to overcome the effects of toxic relationships.

Keith L. Belvin

So, get ready for a transformative journey as you dive into the pages of this book. Allow Keith's story and guidance to inspire and motivate you to create the life you truly deserve – a life free from the chains of toxicity and filled with love, happiness, and healthy relationships.

Let's take those first steps toward healing because you deserve nothing less!

Yolanda Marie Tate
US Army Retired, IT Professional, Wellness Consultant, and Coach
Owner, Elevate 2 Wellness, LLC
www.elevate2wellness.c

12 Steps to Recovering from A Toxic Relationship

Self-Assessment Quiz: Identifying Toxic Patterns

Before reading the book, please take a minute to assess what type of relationship you were or are currently in.

In this section titled **"Self-Assessment Quiz: Identifying Toxic Patterns,"** I wanted to provide readers with a valuable tool for gaining insight into their behaviors and identifying potential toxic patterns in their relationships. As a Crisis Specialist, my personal development expertise and experience as a counselor and life coach shine through in this chapter as he presents a comprehensive quiz to help you better understand tendencies and behaviors. By taking this quiz and reflecting on your responses, readers can better understand themselves and their relationship patterns, which can be an essential first step in creating healthier, more fulfilling relationships. Through thoughtful and insightful guidance, I pray this assessment empowers readers to take ownership of their behaviors and actively work towards building more positive relationships in their lives.

<u>Here's the self-assessment quiz that will identify toxic patterns in your relationships and evaluate the level of toxicity:</u>

Instructions: Answer each question with a **"Yes"** or **"No"** response. Be honest with yourself and try to answer each question to the best of your ability.

Does your partner criticize or belittle you publicly or privately?

Does your partner blame you for their problems or bad mood?

Does your partner isolate you from your friends and family?

Does your partner try to control your actions, decisions, or choices?

Does your partner threaten you with physical or emotional violence or use physical force to control you?

Does your partner constantly monitor your phone, emails, or social media accounts?

Does your partner consistently invalidate your feelings or emotions?

Does your partner use guilt or shame to control you?

Does your partner manipulate or lie to you?

Does your partner refuse to take responsibility for their actions or apologize when they've done something wrong?

Scoring:

If you answered **"Yes"** to **0-2** questions, your relationship is likely healthy and non-toxic.

12 Steps to Recovering from A Toxic Relationship

If you answered **"Yes"** to **3-5** questions, some toxic patterns in your relationship may need to be addressed.

If you answered **"Yes"** to **6 or more** questions, your relationship is likely very toxic, and you may need professional help to address the situation. If you want to set up a Free Discovery Call with Keith K. L. Belvin, visit https://linktr.ee/keith_kl_belvin. If you would like to take a digital version of the **"Self-Assessment Quiz: Identifying Toxic Patterns."** to be able to print or share, please go to: **https://forms.gle/YX1pvDkaQ4pJXmCG9**

*****Remember, self-assessment quizzes are not a substitute for professional advice or therapy. If you feel like you may be in a toxic relationship, it's essential to seek help from a trusted friend, family member, or mental health professional. Reach out to Keith K. L. Belvin, MHSC, MS Ed, for Counseling Support*****

Keith L. Belvin

Introduction

In our society, relationships are often romanticized as the ultimate goal in life. From a young age, we are taught to seek love and companionship, and we are bombarded with images of happy couples in movies, books, and social media. However, not all relationships are healthy or fulfilling; some can be toxic.

A toxic relationship harms one or both partners, either physically or emotionally. It can take many forms, such as emotional abuse, manipulation, gaslighting, or physical violence. Toxic relationships can be challenging to identify, especially when the abuse is subtle or insidious. But once you realize you are in a toxic relationship, it can be tough to extricate yourself and move on.

"12 Steps to Recovering from A Toxic Relationship" by Keith K. L. Belvin, MHSC, MS Ed, is a guidebook for anyone who has been able to remove themselves from a toxic relationship and is looking to heal and move forward. Belvin draws from his Education, having a master's in human service counseling and another in Education. However, Belvin also relies on his years of experience as a mental health counselor, professional educator, and relationship expert to provide practical, actionable steps readers can take to regain control of their lives and create a healthier, happier future.

The book is divided into twelve chapters, each focusing on a different step in the recovery process.

12 Steps to Recovering from A Toxic Relationship

The efforts are designed to be taken in order, each building on the previous one. Belvin provides clear, concise explanations and sub-steps to each step to help readers implement them in their own lives.

Before starting the recovery process, you must acknowledge that you were in a toxic relationship. This acknowledgment can be difficult, especially if you have been in a relationship for a long time or the abuse has been subtle. Belvin guides you in recognizing the signs of a toxic relationship and overcoming any resistance or denial you may feel. Belvin created an independent assessment that can be taken to help you learn if you are or were in a toxic relationship. You can take the evaluation or pass it on to a friend who may need it by going to; https://bit.ly/12StepsAssessmentForm.

Once you acknowledge you were in a toxic relationship, setting boundaries is next. Accepting this can be challenging, especially if your partner has been controlling or manipulative. Belvin provides practical tips on selecting and sticking to limits, even in the face of resistance or pushback. Other steps in the recovery process include learning to communicate effectively, developing a support system, and creating a vision for your future.

One of the most significant strengths of "12 Steps To Recovering From A Toxic Relationship" is that it is grounded in research and real-world experience. Belvin draws on the latest findings in psychology and neuroscience to explain why toxic relationships are so damaging and how to recover from them. At the same time, he uses real-life examples from his practice to illustrate the concepts and make them accessible to readers.

In addition to its practical advice and real-life examples, "12 Steps To Recovering From A Toxic Relationship" is also written in an engaging, conversational style that makes it easy to read and understand. Belvin is empathetic and non-judgmental, and his tone is supportive and encouraging.

Overall, "12 Steps To Recovering From A Toxic Relationship" is an excellent resource for a person removed from a toxic relationship and looking to move on. Whether you are just starting to acknowledge that your relationship was toxic or on your way to recovery, this book provides practical, actionable advice to help you heal and create a brighter future.

12 Steps to Recovering from A Toxic Relationship

Step 1: Accept Your Current Mental and Emotional Positioning with Your Life

Accepting your current mental and emotional position after getting out of a toxic relationship can be complex and challenging. However, it is essential to healing and moving forward with your life. Here are some steps you can take to accept your current mental and emotional positioning:

Allow yourself to feel your emotions.

Allowing yourself to feel your emotions after getting out of a relationship, particularly a toxic one, is integral to the healing process. Trying to bury or ignore painful emotions to move on quickly can be tempting, but this approach is often counterproductive and can lead to deeper emotional wounds in the long run. Instead, by allowing yourself to feel your emotions, you are acknowledging the depth of your experience and giving yourself permission to grieve and healthily process your feelings.

It is also important to remember that emotions are a natural and necessary part of the human experience. Allowing yourself to feel and express your emotions can help you process and release negative energy, leading to greater emotional clarity and understanding. Additionally, denying or suppressing your emotions can lead to physical symptoms such as headaches, stomach aches, or chronic pain. By allowing yourself to feel your emotions, you are taking an essential step towards your healing and well-being and giving yourself the space and time you need to recover from the effects of a toxic relationship fully.

Take care of your physical health.

Taking care of your physical health after getting out of a relationship, especially a toxic one, is crucial for your overall well-being and recovery. The emotional turmoil and stress that comes with a breakup can take a toll on your physical health, causing symptoms such as fatigue, poor sleep, and decreased immunity. Prioritizing physical self-care can help mitigate these effects and give you the energy and strength to focus on healing.

Some ways to take care of your physical health after a toxic relationship include maintaining a healthy diet, regular exercise, and getting enough rest. Eating a balanced diet can help regulate mood and energy levels, while exercise can help release stress and boost endorphins. Getting enough rest is also vital for both physical and emotional health, as it allows your body to recharge and repair. By prioritizing physical self-care, you are taking care of your body and giving yourself the resources and energy to focus on your emotional healing and recovery.

Practice self-compassion.

After getting out of a relationship, especially a toxic one, practicing self-compassion is essential. Self-compassion means treating yourself with the same kindness, concern, and understanding you would offer to a good friend. It's about acknowledging and accepting your emotions, strengths, and limitations without judgment or self-criticism. Practicing self-compassion can help you cope with the intense emotions and self-doubt often resulting from a breakup. It can also help you cultivate a more positive and supportive relationship with yourself, which is essential for long-term well-being.

To practice self-compassion, start by recognizing and acknowledging your feelings without judgment. This means allowing yourself to feel your emotions, even if they are uncomfortable or painful, without trying to suppress or ignore them. Next, practice self-kindness by offering yourself support, comfort, and encouragement. This might involve speaking to yourself gently and understanding, reminding yourself that making mistakes is okay, or engaging in activities that bring you joy and comfort. Finally, practice mindfulness by staying present and observing your thoughts and emotions without judgment or attachment. This can help you develop a more balanced and realistic perspective on your situation and cultivate greater resilience and inner strength.

Seek support from others.

Getting out of a negative relationship can be a traumatic experience that leaves one feeling alone, vulnerable, and emotionally drained. It is essential to seek support from others during this difficult time. Isolating oneself after a breakup is tempting but can prolong healing and lead to further emotional distress. Individuals can find comfort and understanding by contacting friends, family, or a support group. It is important to remember that it is not a sign of weakness to seek help; instead, it is a sign of strength and self-awareness. A support system can provide a listening ear, validation, and encouragement, which can help one regain a sense of control over their life.

Seeking support can also provide a fresh perspective on the situation. Sometimes, individuals in an antagonistic relationship can become isolated from others, and their views can become skewed. A supportive friend or family member can offer a different viewpoint, which can help process the breakup. Additionally, support can help individuals understand that they are not alone and that others have gone through similar situations. Finally, sharing experiences and feelings with others can foster a sense of community and provide a source of motivation to move forward. Support can come in various forms, including therapy, counseling, support groups, or simply talking to a trusted friend or family member. The key is to find a support system that works for the individual and to be open to receiving help from others.

Set boundaries.

12 Steps to Recovering from A Toxic Relationship

Setting boundaries is essential for maintaining healthy relationships and promoting self-respect. It involves understanding your limits and communicating them clearly to others. After getting out of a negative relationship, it is crucial to set boundaries to avoid falling into similar patterns. You are taking control of your life and relationships by setting boundaries. This means that you get to decide what is acceptable and what is not. In addition, when you set boundaries, you protect your physical and emotional well-being.

Furthermore, setting boundaries helps you to respect yourself and communicate your needs effectively. This process can be complicated, especially if this is the first time you have done it. It requires you to be honest with yourself and others about what you are comfortable with and what you are not. You may also need to be firm in your communication and stand your ground when others push your boundaries. Nevertheless, setting boundaries can lead to healthier and more fulfilling relationships, as people will know where they stand with you and what is expected of them. It also helps to build trust and respect, as people will see that you value yourself and are willing to advocate for your needs.

Seeking support can also provide a fresh perspective on the situation. Sometimes, individuals in an antagonistic relationship can become isolated from others, and their views can become skewed. A supportive friend or family member can offer a different viewpoint, which can help process the breakup. Additionally, support can help individuals understand that they are not alone and that others have gone through similar situations. Finally, sharing experiences and feelings with others can foster a sense of community and provide a source of motivation to move forward. Support can come in various forms, including therapy, counseling, support groups, or simply talking to a trusted friend or family member. The key is to find a support system that works for the individual and to be open to receiving help from others.

Focus on the present.

After getting out of a negative relationship, it can be challenging to let go of the past and move on. However, focusing on the present is essential for healing and moving forward. Dwelling on the past can lead to negative thoughts, anxiety, and depression, impacting a person's overall well-being. Therefore, it is crucial to shift the focus to the present and practice mindfulness to stay grounded and aware of the current moment. This can be done by engaging in activities that bring joy and happiness, practicing meditation or deep breathing exercises, or simply being present in the moment by observing the surroundings and letting go of negative thoughts.

Focusing on the present can also help people identify their needs and set goals to achieve them. When a person is stuck in the past, it can be challenging to identify their current needs and desires. However, by focusing on the present, they can determine what they want and need and take the necessary steps to achieve them. This can lead to empowerment, motivation, and a renewed sense of purpose. In addition, by focusing on the present, a person can also improve their relationships with others and build stronger connections as they become more aware and present in their interactions. Focusing on the present is essential for healing and moving forward after a negative relationship. It allows a person to take control of their life and create a brighter future.

Cultivate gratitude.

After getting out of a toxic relationship, it is crucial to cultivate gratitude as it can help in the healing process and bring a positive shift in one's perspective. A toxic relationship can leave one feeling drained, hurt, and having a negative outlook. Focusing on gratitude can help one shift their attention toward positive aspects of life, leading to joy and contentment. Practicing gratitude can also help one find meaning in their experiences, as it encourages them to reflect on their strengths and accomplishments, which can help rebuild one's self-esteem and confidence. By being grateful for the lessons learned from the toxic relationship, one can transform the experience into an opportunity for growth and personal development.

In addition, cultivating gratitude can also improve one's mental and physical health. Studies have shown that people who practice gratitude regularly experience lower levels of stress, anxiety, and depression. Gratitude can help reduce negative emotions and increase positive emotions, such as happiness and joy.

It can also improve one's relationships with others by promoting empathy, forgiveness, and kindness. By cultivating gratitude, one can create a positive cycle of well-being that can benefit all aspects of their life, including work, family, and personal relationships. Therefore, practicing gratitude after exiting a toxic relationship is essential to promote healing, personal growth, and overall well-being.

Let go of guilt or shame:

Once you have removed yourself from a negative relationship, letting go of guilt or shame is crucial. Holding onto these negative emotions can hinder the healing process and prevent one from moving forward. Guilt and shame are common emotions experienced by survivors of toxic relationships, but it is essential to understand that these feelings are not justified. Unhealthy relationships are often characterized by manipulation, control, and emotional abuse, and it is not the survivor's fault for being in such a relationship. Acknowledging this fact and letting go of guilt and shame, one can take the first step towards healing and rebuilding their self-esteem.

Letting go of guilt and shame can also help one to develop a positive self-image and restore a sense of self-worth. Holding onto these negative emotions can lead to self-blame and feelings of inadequacy, affecting one's mental and emotional well-being. It is crucial to recognize that everyone deserves to be treated with respect and kindness, and no one should ever be made to feel like they are not enough. By letting go of guilt and shame, one can begin to focus on their strengths and accomplishments, leading to a more positive and confident outlook on life. Therefore, releasing guilt and shame after exiting a toxic relationship is essential to promote healing, self-growth, and a positive self-image.

Create a new routine:

Creating a new routine after leaving a toxic relationship is essential to establish a sense of stability and control over one's life. Unhealthy relationships can be characterized by a lack of structure and unpredictability, leading to a loss of routine and stability. Creating a new way can provide a sense of design and order, which can help in the healing process and promote a sense of well-being. In addition, establishing a new routine can also create a sense of control over their life, which can be empowering and liberating.

Creating a new routine can also help one to develop new healthy habits and prioritize self-care. Leaving a toxic relationship can be emotionally and mentally exhausting, and it is crucial to prioritize self-care to promote healing and recovery. By creating a new routine that includes self-care activities such as exercise, meditation, or spending time with loved ones, one can develop new healthy habits that can benefit their mental and physical health. A new routine can also help one to establish boundaries and create a sense of balance in their life, which can be crucial in maintaining healthy relationships and achieving personal goals. Therefore, creating a new routine after leaving a toxic relationship is essential in promoting healing, establishing control, and developing new healthy habits.

Celebrate your progress.

Celebrating progress after leaving a toxic relationship is crucial to acknowledge the efforts and accomplishments made during the healing process. Surviving a toxic relationship is not easy, and it takes a lot of courage, strength, and resilience to leave and move on. However, celebrating progress can help one acknowledge the hard work and effort put into healing and recovery, boosting self-esteem and confidence. It can also help to promote a positive outlook toward the future and encourage further personal growth and development.

Celebrating progress can also help one to develop a sense of closure and move on from the toxic relationship. Toxic relationships can leave one feeling trapped, powerless, and with a sense of hopelessness. Celebrating progress can help one to reclaim their power and take control of their life, which can be liberating and empowering. It can also help one to recognize the positive changes that have occurred since leaving the toxic relationship, which can be motivating and encouraging. Therefore, celebrating progress after leaving a toxic relationship is essential in promoting self-esteem, developing a positive outlook, and moving on from the past.

In addition, celebrating progress can also inspire and motivate others who may be going through a similar experience. Sharing one's progress can help raise awareness about toxic relationships' effects and encourage others to seek help and support. It can also serve as a source of inspiration and hope for those who may feel trapped in a toxic relationship and need the courage to leave. Therefore, celebrating progress not only benefits oneself but can also have a positive impact on others and promote a sense of community and support.

Healing is a journey; recovering from a toxic relationship takes time and effort. However, these steps can help you accept your mental and emotional position and move towards a brighter future. Getting your current mental and emotional positioning after leaving a toxic relationship can be challenging, but it is a necessary step toward healing and moving forward. Remember to be kind and compassionate to yourself, seek support, let go of guilt and shame, focus on the present, and celebrate your progress. With time, patience, and perseverance, you can create a brighter future for yourself.

Step 2: Pay Close Attention To How You Got To This Point

Paying close attention to how you got to this point after getting out of a toxic relationship can help you break the cycle, avoid repeating mistakes, build self-awareness, heal, and move forward, and set goals for the future. It's an essential step in healing and creating positivity for yourself.

Reflect on your past.

Reflecting on the past after leaving a toxic relationship is essential to process and make sense of the experience. Toxic relationships can leave one feeling confused, hurt, and with a sense of uncertainty. Reflecting on the past can help one understand what happened, how it affected them, and how to prevent it from happening again. It can also help one identify patterns and behaviors that may have contributed to the toxic relationship, which can be crucial in preventing similar situations.

Reflecting on the past can also help one to release negative emotions and find closure. Toxic relationships can leave a trail of emotional scars, and it is essential to acknowledge and process these emotions to promote healing and recovery. Reflecting on the past can help one to confront and release negative emotions such as anger, sadness, and hurt, which can be cathartic and healing. It can also help one to find closure and move on from the past, which can be empowering and liberating. Therefore, reflecting on the past after leaving a toxic relationship is essential in promoting understanding, identifying patterns, releasing negative emotions, and finding closure.

In addition, reflecting on the past can also help one to grow and learn from the experience. Leaving a toxic relationship can be a turning point in one's life, and it is crucial to take the opportunity to reflect on the knowledge and learn from it. Reflecting on the past can help one to identify their strengths and weaknesses, develop new coping mechanisms, and establish healthy boundaries. It can also help one to learn about themselves and what they want and need from future relationships, which can be crucial in building healthy and fulfilling relationships. Therefore, reflecting on the past promotes healing and closure and can lead to personal growth and development.

Identify your triggers.

Identifying your triggers after leaving a toxic relationship is essential to avoid falling back into old patterns and behaviors. Toxic relationships can leave deep emotional scars, and it is not uncommon for individuals to develop triggers that can lead to adverse emotional reactions and behaviors. Identifying your triggers can help you to recognize situations or events that may trigger negative emotions, such as fear, anxiety, or anger, which can be crucial in preventing relapse into a toxic relationship. It can also help you to develop new coping mechanisms and strategies to manage your triggers, which can be beneficial in promoting emotional and mental well-being.

Identifying your triggers can also help you to establish healthy boundaries and prioritize self-care. Toxic relationships can blur boundaries and lead to self-identity loss, harming emotional and mental health. Identifying your triggers can help you establish healthy boundaries and identify situations or people that may harm your emotional well-being. It can also help you to prioritize self-care by developing new healthy habits and activities that promote emotional and mental well-being. Therefore, identifying your triggers after leaving a toxic relationship is essential in preventing relapse, promoting emotional and mental well-being, and establishing healthy boundaries.

In addition, identifying your triggers can also help you to communicate your needs effectively and build healthy relationships. Toxic relationships can make it difficult for individuals to communicate their needs effectively, leading to a breakdown in communication and trust. Identifying your triggers can help you understand and share your needs effectively with others, which can be crucial in building healthy and fulfilling relationships. It can also help you to recognize when a relationship is not healthy or safe and take steps to end it, which can be empowering and liberating. Therefore, identifying your triggers not only benefits oneself but can also lead to the development of healthy and fulfilling relationships.

<u>Assess your boundaries.</u>

Assessing your boundaries after leaving a toxic relationship is essential to establish a sense of self-worth, protecting your emotional well-being, and ensuring healthy relationships moving forward. Unhealthy relationships often violate personal boundaries, leaving individuals powerless and without a clear understanding of their needs and limits. Assessing your limitations allows you to regain control over your life and define what is acceptable and unacceptable in your relationships. In addition, it lets you set clear limits on how others can treat you and helps you communicate your needs effectively.

By assessing your boundaries, you can also prevent future toxic relationships from occurring. Understanding and defining your limits allows you to recognize early warning signs and red flags. It empowers you to make informed decisions about who you allow into your life and sets the standard for the treatment you deserve. Assessing your boundaries helps prioritize your well-being and teaches others how to treat you respectfully and kindly. It creates a healthier relationship dynamic, promoting mutual understanding and fostering a sense of safety and trust.

Moreover, assessing your boundaries after leaving a toxic relationship promotes self-growth and personal development. It allows self-reflection and introspection, allowing you to identify areas where your borders may have been compromised or neglected. By assessing your boundaries, you can determine what values and behaviors align with your authentic self. It allows you to reevaluate your needs and desires and make choices that align with your personal growth and happiness. Setting boundaries establishes a solid foundation for future relationships based on mutual respect, trust, and healthy boundaries.

Review your communication style.

Reviewing your communication style after leaving a toxic relationship is crucial to regain control over your voice, enhance healthy interactions, and rebuilding trust in relationships. Toxic relationships often involve patterns of manipulation, gaslighting, and unhealthy communication dynamics. Therefore, it is essential to reflect on your communication style and identify any negative habits or behaviors that may have developed. Reviewing your communication style, you can become aware of any tendencies to withhold your thoughts and emotions or engage in passive-aggressive behaviors. This self-awareness allows you to consciously improve your communication skills, express yourself authentically, and effectively assert your needs and boundaries.

Moreover, reviewing your communication style helps you rebuild trust and develop healthier connections with others. Toxic relationships can erode trust and make establishing open and honest communication with new partners, friends, or family members challenging. By assessing your communication style, you can identify any lingering behaviors or triggers that hinder open dialogue and connection. It provides an opportunity to address any tendencies to become defensive, dismissive, or overly accommodating. By practicing effective and respectful communication, such as active listening, expressing empathy, and using strong language, you can foster trust, build healthier relationships, and create an environment of mutual understanding and respect. Reviewing your communication style is essential in nurturing positive connections and establishing healthy communication patterns.

Explore your values.

Exploring your values after leaving a toxic relationship is essential for rediscovering your sense of self, aligning with your authentic desires, and establishing fulfilling relationships in the future. Unhealthy relationships often compromise or suppress one's values, leading to a loss of personal identity and a sense of disconnection. You can reconnect with your core beliefs, principles, and aspirations by exploring your values. This exploration allows you to understand what truly matters to you and what brings you joy and fulfillment. It empowers you to make choices that align with your values and build a life that reflects your true self. Furthermore, exploring your values lets you set healthy boundaries and make informed relationship decisions. Understanding your values helps establish a solid foundation for romantic, friendship, or professional connections. By knowing your values, you can identify and attract individuals with similar beliefs and principles, fostering meaningful and supportive connections. It also helps you recognize any misalignments or red flags in relationships early on, allowing you to make choices that prioritize your well-being and prevent toxic dynamics from repeating. Finally, exploring your values after leaving a toxic relationship is vital to creating a fulfilling and authentic life built on your terms.

Evaluate your self-esteem.

Evaluating your self-esteem after leaving a toxic relationship is essential for rebuilding your sense of self-worth, regaining confidence, and cultivating a healthy self-image. Unhealthy relationships often involve emotional abuse, manipulation, and constant criticism that can significantly damage your self-esteem. Therefore, it is essential to take the time to evaluate your self-esteem and assess the impact the toxic relationship had on your self-perception. By doing so, you can identify any negative beliefs or internalized criticisms that may have developed and work towards challenging and replacing them with more positive and empowering thoughts.

Evaluating your self-esteem also allows you to prioritize self-care and focus on your well-being. Toxic relationships often prioritize the needs and desires of the toxic partner, leaving little room for self-care and self-nurturing. By evaluating your self-esteem, you can identify areas where you may have neglected your needs or compromised your well-being. This evaluation serves as a reminder to prioritize self-love, self-compassion, and self-care moving forward. It helps you cultivate a healthy relationship with yourself, promoting emotional resilience and creating a solid foundation for future relationships based on mutual respect and care. Evaluating your self-esteem after leaving a toxic relationship is essential in reclaiming your power and building a positive self-image.

Analyze your support system.

Analyzing your support system after leaving a toxic relationship is crucial for building a solid network of individuals who provide love, understanding, and emotional support. Unfortunately, toxic relationships often isolate individuals, resulting in a diminished support system. By analyzing your support system, you can assess who has been there for you during difficult times and who you can rely on for guidance, validation, and encouragement. In addition, this analysis helps you identify the people who genuinely care about your well-being and are willing to provide the support you need as you heal and rebuild your life.

Analyzing your support system also allows you to identify toxic or unsupportive individuals who may hinder your progress. In some cases, individuals from your previous poisonous relationship may attempt to maintain control or manipulate you even after the relationship ends. By evaluating your support system, you can recognize any negative influences and take steps to distance yourself from individuals who perpetuate toxic behaviors. Surrounding yourself with positive and supportive people who uplift and empower you is essential for your healing journey. It creates a nurturing environment that fosters growth, provides validation, and reinforces the worthiness of healthy and respectful relationships. Analyzing your support system is crucial in building a solid foundation of support and ensuring your emotional well-being as you move forward.

Reflect on your decision-making process.

Reflecting on your decision-making process after leaving a toxic relationship is essential for developing self-awareness, building resilience, and making healthier choices in the future. Unhealthy relationships often involve a pattern of control, manipulation, and decision-making that prioritizes the needs and desires of the toxic partner over your own. Reflecting on your decision-making process allows you to examine any patterns or tendencies contributing to your involvement in the toxic relationship. In addition, this reflection helps you identify any underlying issues that may have influenced your decision-making, such as low self-esteem, codependency, or fear of being alone. By understanding these patterns, you can actively work towards breaking them and developing a more empowered and autonomous decision-making process.

Reflecting on your decision-making process also enables you to cultivate self-trust and make choices that align with your values and well-being. Toxic relationships can erode your confidence in decision-making and leave you questioning your judgment. By reflecting on your decision-making process, you can assess the impact of the toxic relationship on your ability to trust yourself and regain confidence in your decision-making abilities. This reflection allows you to recognize your strengths and develop a sense of self-trust, essential for making healthier choices in relationships, careers, and other areas of life. It also helps you become more aware of red flags, set clear boundaries, and prioritize your needs and desires when making decisions. Reflecting on your decision-making process is an important step towards reclaiming your autonomy, developing self-trust, and creating a future filled with choices that empower and uplift you.

Keith L. Belvin

Assess your coping mechanisms:

Assessing your coping mechanisms after leaving a toxic relationship is crucial for promoting emotional healing, building resilience, and developing healthier ways of managing stress and adversity. Toxic relationships can take a toll on your mental and emotional well-being, often leading to the development of unhealthy coping mechanisms such as avoidance, numbing, or self-destructive behaviors. By assessing your coping mechanisms, you can gain insight into how you have dealt with the pain and trauma caused by the toxic relationship. In addition, this self-reflection allows you to identify harmful coping strategies and understand their impact on your well-being.

Assessing your coping mechanisms also provides an opportunity for growth and transformation. After leaving a toxic relationship, replacing unhealthy coping mechanisms with healthier alternatives that support your emotional healing and development is essential. By evaluating your coping mechanisms, you can identify areas where you may need professional help or support from trusted individuals. This assessment helps you actively engage in self-care practices, such as therapy, meditation, journaling, or hobbies and activities that bring joy and peace. Developing healthy coping mechanisms allows you to navigate future challenges and triggers with resilience and self-compassion. It empowers you to break free from the cycle of toxicity and create a healthier and more fulfilling life moving forward. Assessing your coping mechanisms is vital in your healing journey and sets the foundation for emotional well-being and personal growth.

Set goals for the future:

Setting goals for the future after leaving a toxic relationship is essential for reclaiming your sense of purpose, creating a positive vision for yourself, and moving forward with intention and determination. Unhealthy relationships often leave individuals feeling depleted, lost, and uncertain about their future. By setting goals, you can regain control and direction in your life. In addition, these goals serve as a roadmap for your growth, allowing you to focus on what you want to achieve and work towards building a life that aligns with your aspirations and values.

Setting goals for the future also empowers you to break free from the past and create a fresh start. It allows you to shift your focus from the toxic relationship and its adverse effects towards building a brighter future. By setting goals, you can channel your energy and resources towards personal development, career advancement, or any other areas of life that hold significance to you. Plans provide a sense of purpose and motivation, propelling you forward and reminding you of your resilience and strength. They help you create a new narrative for yourself, one that is centered around growth, happiness, and personal fulfillment.

Setting goals after leaving a toxic relationship is essential to creating the life you deserve and embracing a future filled with possibilities.

Moreover, setting goals after leaving a toxic relationship promotes self-belief and confidence. Toxic relationships can erode your self-esteem and make you doubt your abilities. Setting achievable goals provides opportunities to prove that you are capable, resilient, and deserving of success. Each goal accomplished becomes a steppingstone towards rebuilding your confidence and developing a positive self-image. As you achieve your goals, whether big or small, you reinforce your belief in your capabilities and strengthen your self-worth. Setting goals for the future empowers you to take ownership of your life and creates a sense of empowerment and agency. It allows you to redefine your identity outside of the toxic relationship and embrace your potential for growth and fulfillment.

Taking responsibility for your growth and healing after a toxic relationship is essential. By paying close attention to how you got to this point, you can learn from your past experiences and create a brighter future. The idea of how you got to this point after getting out of a toxic relationship emphasizes the importance of self-reflection and taking responsibility for your past experiences. By examining the patterns and behaviors that led to the toxic relationship, you can identify any underlying issues that may have contributed to it and work on addressing them. This process can be complex, but it can ultimately help you

12 Steps to Recovering from A Toxic Relationship

avoid similar situations in the future and make healthier relationship choices moving forward. Acknowledging your role in the relationship and focusing on personal growth and healing can create a positive and fulfilling future for yourself.

Keith L. Belvin

Step 3: Don't Blame Yourself For Your Part In The Toxic Relationship

Blaming oneself for their role in a toxic relationship can damage one's mental health and well-being. It's important to remember that both parties contribute to the dysfunction of a toxic relationship. Unhealthy relationships are often characterized by patterns of manipulation, control, and emotional abuse, which are beyond the victim's control. Blaming oneself for these issues can lead to guilt, shame, and low self-esteem, making it difficult to move on and heal. Therefore, it's essential to focus on identifying and addressing the toxic behaviors in the relationship and setting healthy boundaries for oneself rather than placing all the blame on oneself. By doing so, individuals can take steps towards healing and creating healthy relationships in the future.

Acknowledge that relationships involve two people.

Acknowledging that relationships involve two people after leaving a toxic relationship is crucial for personal growth, gaining perspective, and breaking free from a victim mentality. In a toxic relationship, it is common for one person to shoulder the blame and internalize all the responsibility for the toxicity. However, it is essential to recognize that toxic dynamics result from the interaction between both individuals involved. Therefore, you can release blame and cultivate a healthier mindset by acknowledging shared responsibility.

Acknowledging the role of both individuals in a relationship empowers you to take ownership of your actions and choices. It allows you to reflect on your behavior, attitudes, and responses within the toxic relationship. By acknowledging your contribution to the dynamics, you can identify any patterns, codependent behaviors, or unhealthy communication styles you may have developed. This self-reflection provides personal growth and learning opportunities, enabling you to break free from negative patterns and develop healthier relationship skills.

Furthermore, acknowledging that relationships involve two people promotes empathy and understanding. It helps you recognize that the toxic behavior of the other person may have stemmed from unresolved issues, insecurities, or past traumas. This acknowledgment doesn't excuse their behavior but gives you a broader perspective. It can foster compassion and forgiveness, not necessarily for the other person, but for yourself. It lets you let go of resentment and anger, freeing up space for healing and moving forward.

Additionally, acknowledging the shared responsibility in relationships helps you set healthy boundaries and establish more precise communication in future relationships. By recognizing that both individuals contribute to the relationship dynamics, you can establish boundaries that protect your well-being and prevent the repetition of toxic patterns. It enables you to communicate assertively and openly, expressing your needs and concerns while listening to and respecting the other person's needs. Acknowledging the shared responsibility in relationships paves the way for healthier and more balanced connections, where both individuals are accountable for their actions and work together to foster a supportive and nurturing partnership.

Practice self-compassion,

Practicing self-compassion after leaving a toxic relationship is essential for healing, rebuilding self-esteem, and fostering emotional well-being. Unhealthy relationships often leave individuals feeling depleted, unworthy, and full of self-blame. Self-compassion allows you to treat yourself with kindness, understanding, and empathy during this vulnerable time. By practicing self-compassion, you acknowledge and validate your pain, emotions, and experiences without judgment or self-criticism.

Self-compassion provides a nurturing space for healing and self-reflection. It helps you release the guilt and shame that may have been instilled during the toxic relationship. You can reframe negative self-talk and replace it with self-acceptance and self-love through self-compassion. It allows you to embrace your imperfections and recognize that you deserve compassion, care, and understanding, just like anyone else. Self-compassion helps you build resilience and overcome the adverse effects of toxic relationships, allowing you to move forward with a renewed sense of self-worth.

Moreover, practicing self-compassion encourages self-care and prioritizes your well-being. Toxic relationships often neglect individual needs and focus solely on the needs of the toxic partner. By practicing self-compassion, you shift the focus back to yourself and your healing journey. It involves taking care of your physical, emotional, and mental health by engaging in activities that bring you joy, seeking therapy or support, and setting boundaries that protect your well-being. Self-compassion enables you to recognize the importance of self-care and self-nurturing, promoting overall emotional well-being and empowering you to create a life aligned with your values and desires.

Furthermore, practicing self-compassion cultivates a positive and forgiving mindset. It lets you let go of self-blame and forgive yourself for any perceived mistakes or shortcomings. Self-compassion acknowledges that you did the best you could with the resources and knowledge you had at the time. Practicing self-compassion frees you from resentment, anger, or guilt. It creates space for personal growth and transformation, enabling you to develop a healthier self-image and establish more beneficial relationships. Practicing self-compassion is essential in rebuilding your life after a toxic relationship, fostering self-acceptance, and creating a foundation of love and compassion for yourself.

Reflect on your role in the relationship.

Reflecting on your role in the toxic relationship after leaving is essential for self-awareness, personal growth, and breaking negative patterns. It allows you to gain insight into the dynamics contributing to the toxicity and take responsibility for your actions. Self-reflection enables you to examine your behavior, attitudes, and choices within the relationship, acknowledging any patterns or tendencies that may have perpetuated the toxicity. By reflecting on your role, you can identify codependent behaviors, enabling you to address them and develop healthier relationship skills.

Reflecting on your role also helps you heal and overcome guilt or self-blame. Toxic relationships often lead individuals to question their worth and internalize the blame for the dysfunction. However, through reflection, you can gain a more objective perspective on the dynamics and recognize that both parties contribute to the relationship's dynamics. This realization allows you to release unnecessary guilt or self-blame and focus on healing. In addition, reflecting on your role enables you to forgive yourself for mistakes or perceived shortcomings, fostering self-compassion and creating space for growth and self-improvement.

Additionally, reflecting on your role in the toxic relationship empowers you to break negative patterns and establish healthier boundaries and communication in future relationships. By acknowledging your part in the toxic dynamic, you become aware of any enabling behaviors, self-sacrifice, or lack of assertiveness that may have contributed to the toxicity. This awareness allows you to set healthier boundaries that protect your well-being and prevent the repetition of toxic patterns. It also lets you develop practical communication skills, ensuring your needs and concerns are expressed respectfully and assertively. Finally, reflecting on your role in the relationship provides an opportunity for personal growth, helping you establish healthier relationship dynamics and create a future filled with more fulfilling and mutually supportive connections.

Accept that you cannot control the other person.

Accepting that you cannot control the other person in a toxic relationship is essential for finding peace, letting go of resentment, and embracing personal growth. In a toxic relationship, it is common to have a strong desire to change or control the behavior of the tainted individual. However, accepting that you cannot control someone else's actions or choices allows you to shift your focus inward and reclaim your power. In addition, it frees you from the exhausting and futile cycle of trying to change someone unwilling or unable to.

Acceptance promotes emotional healing and lets you let go of resentment and anger. When you acknowledge that you cannot control the other person's behavior, you release yourself from responsibility for their actions. This acceptance allows you to redirect your energy toward healing and personal growth. It enables you to process your emotions and work through any lingering pain or trauma caused by the toxic relationship. Accepting that you cannot control the other person opens the door to forgiveness, both for them and yourself, freeing you from the emotional weight of the past.

Furthermore, accepting your lack of control fosters self-compassion and self-acceptance. It helps you recognize that you did the best you could in a difficult situation and that it is not your fault for the toxic behavior of the other person. This acceptance allows you to let go of self-blame and judgment. It enables you to be kind to yourself and acknowledge your own worth and value independent of the actions of others. Accepting that you cannot control the other person cultivates a sense of self-empowerment as you take ownership of your choices and focus on creating a healthier and more fulfilling future.

Moreover, accepting your lack of control promotes personal growth and resilience. It allows you to reflect on the lessons learned from the toxic relationship and use them as steppingstones for personal development. By accepting that you cannot control the other person, you recognize the importance of establishing healthy boundaries, prioritizing your well-being, and surrounding yourself with supportive and respectful relationships. This acceptance empowers you to make choices that align with your values and desires, paving the way for a future filled with healthier and more fulfilling connections. It fosters resilience as you learn from the past and move forward with newfound strength and wisdom. Accepting your lack of control is essential to embracing personal growth, finding inner peace, and creating a life free from the toxicity of trying to change others.

Seek feedback from trusted friends and family.

Seeking feedback from trusted friends and family after leaving a toxic relationship is essential for gaining perspective, validating your experiences, and rebuilding trust in relationships. Toxic relationships often manipulate individuals into doubting their judgment and perceptions. Seeking feedback from trusted loved ones allows you to gain an outside perspective on the dynamics of the toxic relationship. Their insights and observations can provide validation and confirmation of your experiences, helping you break free from the gaslighting and manipulation that may have occurred. It empowers you to trust your perceptions and regain confidence in assessing healthy and unhealthy relationship dynamics.

Furthermore, seeking feedback from trusted friends and family helps heal. Sharing your experiences and emotions with loved ones who genuinely care about your well-being creates a support system that nurtures your emotional recovery. Opening up and seeking feedback allows others to provide empathy, understanding, and validation, which can be incredibly healing. Their feedback can offer comfort, reassurance, and solidarity, reminding you that you are not alone. It also helps you process your emotions and gain clarity as you navigate the aftermath of the toxic relationship. Seeking feedback from trusted individuals provides a safe space to express your feelings, seek guidance, and receive the support you need to heal and move forward.

Additionally, seeking feedback from trusted friends and family helps establish healthier relationship dynamics moving forward. Their feedback can illuminate any red flags or patterns they may have noticed in the toxic relationship. By listening to their observations and insights, you can gain valuable information to help you identify and avoid similar unhealthy dynamics in future relationships. Their feedback can guide setting boundaries, developing practical communication skills, and choosing healthier partners. Seeking feedback from trusted individuals promotes self-awareness and growth, allowing you to build more beneficial relationships based on trust, respect, and mutual support.

Seeking feedback from trusted friends and family after leaving a toxic relationship is crucial for gaining perspective, healing, and establishing healthier relationship dynamics. Their insights and observations provide validation, support, and guidance as you navigate the aftermath of the toxic relationship. By seeking feedback, you empower yourself to trust your perceptions, process your emotions, and rebuild trust in relationships. It is an essential step in your journey towards healing, growth, and creating a future filled with healthy and fulfilling connections.

12 Steps to Recovering from A Toxic Relationship

Focus on your personal growth.

Focusing on personal growth after leaving a toxic relationship is essential for rebuilding self-esteem, establishing healthy boundaries, and creating a fulfilling and empowered life. Toxic relationships can leave individuals feeling diminished, unworthy, and emotionally drained. You prioritize your well-being and development by shifting the focus to personal growth. It allows you to invest time and energy in self-improvement, fostering a sense of empowerment and self-worth.

Engaging in personal growth after a toxic relationship helps rebuild self-esteem that may have been eroded during the toxic dynamics. It involves nurturing self-compassion, self-acceptance, and self-love. You actively build a positive self-image by engaging in activities promoting self-care, setting achievable goals, and seeking personal development opportunities. Personal growth empowers you to challenge negative beliefs and replace them with empowering and affirming ones. It enables you to recognize your strengths, talents, and worth, fostering a renewed sense of confidence and self-esteem.

Furthermore, focusing on personal growth allows you to establish and maintain healthy boundaries in future relationships. Toxic relationships often blur boundaries and disregard individual needs and limits. You better understand your values, priorities, and limitations by engaging in personal development. This self-awareness enables you to establish clear and healthy boundaries that protect your emotional, physical, and mental well-being. In addition, it empowers you to communicate assertively and advocate for your needs, fostering relationships based on respect and mutual support.

Moreover, focusing on personal growth provides an opportunity for self-discovery and creating a fulfilling life aligned with your authentic self. After leaving a toxic relationship, you can explore your interests, passions, and dreams without the constraints of toxic dynamics. Personal growth involves self-reflection, setting goals, and pursuing activities that bring joy and fulfillment. It allows you to identify your values, desires, and aspirations and make choices that align with them. By focusing on personal growth, you cultivate a sense of purpose, independence, and fulfillment, creating a life that reflects your true self and brings you happiness and satisfaction.

Focusing on personal growth after leaving a toxic relationship is essential for rebuilding self-esteem, establishing healthy boundaries, and creating a fulfilling life. It enables you to prioritize your well-being and development, fostering a sense of empowerment and self-worth. You rebuild self-esteem, establish healthy boundaries, and discover your authentic self through personal growth. It is a transformative journey that allows you to heal from toxic relationships, embrace your strengths, and create a future filled with self-fulfillment and happiness.

12 Steps to Recovering from A Toxic Relationship

Let go of guilt and shame.

Letting go of guilt and shame after leaving a toxic relationship is essential for healing, self-acceptance, and reclaiming your emotional well-being. In toxic relationships, manipulative tactics and emotional abuse often lead individuals to internalize feelings of guilt and shame, blaming themselves for the dysfunction. However, it is crucial to recognize that the toxicity in the relationship was not your fault. Letting go of guilt and shame allows you to release responsibility for the toxic dynamics and shift the focus toward your healing and growth.

By letting go of guilt and shame, you create space for self-compassion and self-forgiveness. Toxic relationships often erode self-esteem and leave individuals feeling unworthy and flawed. However, it is essential to acknowledge that no one is perfect, and mistakes or shortcomings do not justify mistreatment. Self-compassion involves treating yourself with kindness and understanding and recognizing that you deserve love and respect regardless of past experiences. It allows you to forgive yourself for any perceived mistakes or choices made in the toxic relationship and embrace a mindset of self-acceptance and self-love.

Letting go of guilt and shame also enables you to break free from the cycle of self-blame and self-judgment. Toxic relationships can instill a sense of inadequacy and a belief that you are at fault for the toxicity. However, realizing that you are not responsible for someone else's actions or choices is essential. By releasing guilt and shame, you reclaim your power and agency, recognizing that you can prioritize your well-being and happiness. It empowers you to let go of the negative beliefs and internalized blame, freeing yourself from the emotional weight that may have held you back. Letting go of guilt and shame opens the door to personal growth, allowing you to move forward with a renewed sense of self-worth and a clear vision for a healthier and more fulfilling future.

Releasing guilt and shame after leaving a toxic relationship is essential for healing, self-acceptance, and reclaiming your emotional well-being. It involves recognizing that the toxic dynamics were not your fault and practicing self-compassion and self-forgiveness. By letting go of guilt and shame, you break free from the cycle of self-blame and self-judgment, empowering yourself to prioritize your well-being and create a future filled with self-love and happiness. It is a transformative process that allows you to embrace your worth, release the weight of the past, and step into a new chapter of your life with confidence and resilience.

Avoid self-blame and negative self-talk.

Avoiding self-blame and negative self-talk after leaving a toxic relationship is essential for healing, self-esteem, and cultivating a positive self-image. Toxic relationships often lead to individuals internalizing blame for the dysfunction and mistreatment they experienced. However, it is essential to recognize that the toxicity was not your fault. Avoiding self-blame allows you to let go of unnecessary guilt and shame, paving the way for self-compassion and self-love.

Negative self-talk can be detrimental to your emotional well-being and self-esteem. When you engage in self-blame and negative self-talk, you reinforce negative beliefs about yourself, such as feeling unworthy or deserving of mistreatment. This damaging internal dialogue can hinder your healing process and prevent you from moving forward. Instead, practicing self-compassion and self-acceptance helps you counter negative self-talk. By treating yourself with kindness and understanding, you replace self-blame with self-empowerment and create a nurturing environment for personal growth and self-esteem.

Avoiding self-blame and negative self-talk allows you to reclaim your identity and establish a positive self-image. Toxic relationships can erode self-esteem and distort your perception of self-worth. However, you can rebuild a positive self-image by reframing your thoughts and focusing on your strengths, achievements, and positive qualities. Recognize that you are not defined by the toxic relationship or the negative experiences you endured. Embracing self-acceptance and self-love lets you let go of the toxic narrative and create a new story highlighting your resilience, growth, and inner strength.

Avoiding self-blame and negative self-talk after leaving a toxic relationship is essential for healing, self-esteem, and cultivating a positive self-image. It involves recognizing that the toxicity was not your fault and letting go of unnecessary guilt and shame. By practicing self-compassion and self-acceptance, you counter negative self-talk and create a nurturing environment for personal growth and self-esteem. Avoiding self-blame allows you to reclaim your identity, establish a positive self-image, and move forward with a renewed sense of empowerment and self-worth.

Take responsibility for your part, but don't take on all the blame.

Taking responsibility for your part but not taking on all the blame after leaving a toxic relationship is essential for personal growth, self-forgiveness, and establishing healthy boundaries. Acknowledging your role in the toxic dynamics is an important step towards self-awareness and learning from the experience. By taking responsibility for your part, you can reflect on your behaviors, choices, and patterns that may have contributed to the toxicity. This self-reflection allows you to grow and develop healthier relationship skills moving forward.

However, it is crucial not to take on all the blame for the toxicity in the relationship. Toxic relationships involve the actions and choices of both individuals involved. Blaming yourself entirely can perpetuate guilt, shame, and low self-esteem. It is important to recognize that toxic dynamics result from the interaction between two people, and both parties bear responsibility for their actions. Taking on all the blame can hinder your healing process and prevent you from moving forward.

12 Steps to Recovering from A Toxic Relationship

It is essential to separate your responsibility from the toxic behavior of the other person and understand that you cannot control or change their actions.

Taking responsibility for your part while not shouldering all the blame allows you to practice self-forgiveness and let go of unnecessary guilt. Recognizing your contribution to the toxic relationship is not about self-condemnation but learning and growth. It involves acknowledging enabling behaviors, lack of boundaries, or patterns you need to address and improve upon. By taking responsibility without taking on all the blame, you create space for self-compassion and self-acceptance. This self-forgiveness is crucial for your emotional well-being and allows you to move forward with a renewed sense of empowerment and self-worth.

Taking responsibility for your part but not taking on all the blame after leaving a toxic relationship is essential for personal growth, self-forgiveness, and establishing healthy boundaries. It involves reflecting on your behaviors and patterns while recognizing that the toxicity resulted from the interaction between two people. By taking responsibility, you learn and grow from the experience and protect yourself from unnecessary guilt and self-blame. It is a balancing act that allows you to take ownership of your actions, foster self-compassion, and create a future filled with healthier and more fulfilling relationships.

Move forward with a positive attitude:

Moving forward positively after leaving a toxic relationship is essential for personal growth, resilience, and a happier and healthier future. A positive attitude enables you to shift your focus from the past and embrace the possibilities that lie ahead. It allows you to approach life with optimism, even in the face of challenges and cultivates a mindset of growth and empowerment.

Choosing a positive attitude after leaving a toxic relationship is a powerful tool for personal growth. It enables you to view the experience as a valuable lesson and an opportunity for self-reflection and self-improvement. By maintaining a positive attitude, you can extract wisdom from the past and use it to shape a brighter future. It helps you identify your desired qualities in healthy relationships and set higher standards. A positive attitude makes you more likely to attract positive experiences and nurturing connections, creating a positive cycle of growth and fulfillment.

Furthermore, a positive attitude fosters resilience in the face of adversity. Leaving a toxic relationship can be emotionally challenging, and it is natural to encounter setbacks and obstacles along the way. However, a positive attitude allows you to approach these challenges with determination and optimism. It helps you bounce back, learn from setbacks, and keep moving forward. With a positive mindset, you can navigate the healing process with greater strength and resilience, knowing you can create a better life for yourself.

12 Steps to Recovering from A Toxic Relationship

Moreover, a positive attitude creates a happier and healthier future. Toxic relationships can leave individuals feeling drained, discouraged, and doubting their worth. However, by adopting a positive attitude, you reclaim your power and the belief that you deserve happiness and fulfillment. It opens the door to new opportunities, healthier relationships, and personal satisfaction. A positive attitude allows you to set goals, pursue your passions, and make choices that align with your values and aspirations. It propels you toward a future filled with joy, self-fulfillment, and meaningful connections. Moving forward positively after leaving a toxic relationship is essential for personal growth, resilience, and a brighter future. It enables you to view the past as an opportunity for growth and learning, fostering a mindset of empowerment and self-improvement. With a positive attitude, you can navigate challenges resiliently and bounce back from setbacks. It also sets the stage for creating a happier and healthier future, as it empowers you to set higher standards, attract positive experiences, and live a life that aligns with your values and aspirations. Embracing a positive attitude is a transformative step towards healing, growth, and creating a life filled with positivity and fulfillment. It is essential not to blame yourself for your part in a toxic relationship because blame only perpetuates feelings of guilt, shame, and self-criticism. Toxic relationships involve a complex interplay of dynamics and often result from a combination of factors from both individuals involved. Blaming yourself undermines your self-worth and hinders the healing process necessary for moving forward.

Instead of blaming yourself, focusing on self-reflection and personal growth is more productive. Recognizing your role in the toxic relationship allows you to gain insight into patterns, behaviors, or choices that may need addressing. This self-reflection is not about self-condemnation but learning from experience and positively changing future relationships. By reframing your perspective and accepting that toxicity was not solely your responsibility, you can shift towards a healthier mindset and cultivate self-compassion and forgiveness.

Taking responsibility for your part in a toxic relationship while refraining from blame is a transformative step toward healing and personal empowerment. It allows you to embrace self-awareness and learn from past mistakes, fostering personal growth and setting the stage for healthier relationships in the future. In addition, by letting go of blame, you create space for self-acceptance, self-forgiveness, and a positive outlook on your journey of healing and self-discovery.

It's important to remember that while taking responsibility for one's actions in a relationship is healthy and necessary, blaming oneself excessively or unnecessarily can be harmful and prevent personal growth and healing. Therefore, it's important to practice self-compassion and avoid overly blaming oneself for the problems in the relationship.

Step 4: Offer Yourself Patience and Grace

Getting out of a toxic relationship can be a complex and emotional process. To offer yourself patience and grace during a negative relationship, it's crucial to prioritize your healing and well-being. This can involve taking the time to reflect on your feelings, set healthy boundaries, and seek support from loved ones or a therapist. In addition, it's important to practice self-care, engage in positive activities, and forgive yourself for any mistakes you may have made. Finally, it's also crucial to let go of any shame or guilt associated with the toxic relationship and be kind to yourself throughout the healing process.

Recognize that healing takes time.

Recognizing that healing takes time after getting out of a toxic relationship is essential for self-care, emotional recovery, and establishing healthy boundaries. Leaving an unhealthy relationship can leave deep emotional wounds and scars that require time and patience to heal. Understanding and accepting this process is crucial for allowing yourself the space and compassion to recover fully. Healing from the effects of a toxic relationship involves addressing the trauma, rebuilding self-esteem, and re-establishing a sense of trust and safety. These processes cannot be rushed or forced. It is essential to allow yourself to feel and process the emotions that arise, such as grief, anger, or sadness. Recognizing that healing takes time will enable you to be gentle with yourself and acknowledge that healing is a nonlinear journey with ups and downs. It allows you to prioritize self-care and engage in activities that support your emotional well-being, such as therapy, self-reflection, and engaging with supportive communities.

Additionally, recognizing that healing takes time empowers you to establish healthy boundaries and set realistic expectations. Feeling pressure to quickly move on or "get over" the toxic relationship is expected. However, healing is a personal process that varies for each individual. By recognizing that healing takes time, you can honor your timeline and set boundaries to protect yourself from rushing into new relationships or situations that may hinder your recovery. It allows you to focus on your growth, self-discovery, and inner healing without external pressures or judgment.

Recognizing that healing takes time after getting out of a toxic relationship is crucial for self-care, emotional recovery, and establishing healthy boundaries. It involves understanding and accepting that healing is a gradual process that requires patience, self-compassion, and support. By acknowledging the time, it takes to heal, you can prioritize self-care, engage in activities that support your well-being, and establish healthy boundaries. Remember that healing is unique to everyone, and allowing yourself the time and space to heal will lead to a healthier, more empowered, and fulfilling future.

12 Steps to Recovering from A Toxic Relationship

Practice self-care.

Practicing self-care after getting out of a toxic relationship is essential for your overall well-being, recovery, and rebuilding of a healthy sense of self. Unhealthy relationships can affect your mental, emotional, and physical health. Self-care allows you to prioritize your needs, nurture yourself, and regain control over your life.

Self-care is crucial for healing and recovery after a toxic relationship because it provides a space for self-reflection, self-soothing, and self-compassion. It allows you to process the emotions and trauma associated with the toxic relationship. Engaging in activities that promote relaxation, such as meditation, yoga, or journaling, can help you release stress and tension. Setting aside time for self-reflection enables you to gain clarity, make sense of your experiences, and learn from them. Finally, self-compassion plays a significant role in self-care as it involves treating yourself with kindness, understanding, and forgiveness, letting go of self-blame, and embracing self-love.

Furthermore, self-care empowers you to rebuild a healthy sense of self and establish new boundaries. Toxic relationships often erode your self-esteem, self-worth, and personal boundaries. Engaging in self-care activities that boost self-esteem, such as hobbies, setting achievable goals, or practicing positive affirmations, helps you reconnect with your strengths and regain confidence. Taking care of your physical health through exercise, nourishing your body with nutritious food, and getting enough restful sleep supports your overall well-being. It reinforces the message that you are worthy of care and deserving of a healthy and fulfilling life.

Practicing self-care after exiting a toxic relationship is crucial for your well-being, recovery, and rebuilding a healthy sense of self. It allows you to prioritize your needs, nurture yourself, and regain control over your life. Self-care provides space for self-reflection, self-soothing, and self-compassion, enabling you to process emotions and trauma, gain clarity, and learn from your experiences. It also empowers you to rebuild self-esteem, establish new boundaries, and embrace a healthier and more fulfilling future. Remember that self-care is not selfish but an essential aspect of your healing journey.

Set boundaries for yourself and others.

Setting boundaries for yourself and others after getting out of a toxic relationship is essential for your well-being and self-respect and for creating healthier relationships. Unhealthy relationships often lack boundaries, leading to manipulation, abuse, and disregard for your needs and values. Setting clear boundaries establishes a framework for healthy interactions and protects you from repeating toxicity patterns.

Setting boundaries is crucial for prioritizing well-being and rebuilding your sense of self. It allows you to define acceptable and unacceptable in your relationships and effectively communicate your needs and limits. This empowers you to create a safe and supportive environment where your emotional, physical, and mental well-being are respected. By setting boundaries, you assert your autonomy and self-respect and send a clear message that you deserve to be treated with kindness, respect, and consideration.

Furthermore, setting boundaries helps you identify red flags and protect yourself from entering into new toxic relationships. By reflecting on your past experiences, you can place the behaviors, dynamics, or situations that were harmful or unhealthy. This self-awareness allows you to establish boundaries that serve as a protective shield against potential toxicity. In addition, it helps you set clear expectations and limits for future relationships, preventing you from falling into patterns that may compromise your well-being.

Setting boundaries for yourself and others after exiting a toxic relationship is essential for your well-being and self-respect and for creating healthier relationships. It allows you to define acceptable and unacceptable, communicate your needs effectively, and create a safe environment. Setting boundaries empowers you to prioritize your well-being, rebuild your sense of self, and protect yourself from repeating toxicity patterns. By establishing clear expectations and limits, you can navigate future relationships with a stronger sense of self and create healthier connections based on mutual respect and consideration. Remember that setting boundaries is a powerful act of self-care and a crucial step toward building a happier and more fulfilling life.

Journal your feelings.

Journaling your feelings after getting out of a toxic relationship is essential for emotional healing, self-reflection, and clarity. Toxic relationships can leave you feeling confused, overwhelmed, and emotionally drained. Journaling provides a safe and private space to express and process these complex emotions, allowing you to make sense of your experiences and facilitate healing.

By journaling your feelings, you allow yourself to explore and validate your emotions. It will enable you to release pent-up anger, sadness, or resentment, providing a cathartic outlet. Writing down your thoughts and feelings helps you better understand your experiences, enabling you to untangle the complexities of the toxic relationship and your reactions to it. It can clarify patterns, triggers, and behaviors that were detrimental to your well-being, helping you identify areas for growth and healing.

Journaling also serves as a form of self-reflection and self-discovery. It allows you to delve into your inner thoughts and beliefs, providing an opportunity for self-exploration and introspection. By reflecting on your feelings and experiences, you can gain insight into your needs, desires, and values. This self-awareness helps you establish a stronger sense of self and make informed decisions about future relationships.

12 Steps to Recovering from A Toxic Relationship

Journaling can also serve as a record of your progress and growth, as you can look back on your entries and witness the positive changes and milestones you've achieved.

Journaling your feelings after getting out of a toxic relationship is essential for emotional healing, self-reflection, and clarity. It provides a safe and private space to express and process complex emotions, allowing for catharsis and validation. Journaling enables you to understand your experiences better, untangled complexities, and identify areas for growth and healing. It serves as a form of self-reflection and self-discovery, helping you establish a stronger sense of self and make informed decisions about future relationships. Remember, journaling is a powerful tool for self-care and self-exploration on your healing and personal growth journey.

Seek support.

Seeking support after getting out of a toxic relationship is essential for healing, validation, and rebuilding your life. Toxic relationships can leave lasting emotional scars and make trusting your judgment challenging. Seeking support from trusted friends, family members, or professionals can give you the validation and guidance you need to navigate the healing process effectively.

Support from others helps you feel heard and validated in your experiences. Talking to someone who listens without judgment can provide a safe space to express your feelings, thoughts, and concerns. It helps you process the trauma and emotions associated with the toxic relationship. Supportive individuals can provide an outside perspective and help you gain clarity and insight into the dynamics of toxic relationships. They can offer reassurance that you made the right decision to leave and remind you of your worth and value.

Seeking professional support, such as therapy or counseling, can be particularly beneficial after leaving a toxic relationship. A therapist can provide you with specialized guidance, tools, and coping strategies to navigate the healing process. They can help you process the trauma, identify patterns, and develop healthier relationship skills. Therapy offers a safe and confidential space to explore your experiences, emotions, and self-growth. A professional can also help you rebuild your self-esteem, set boundaries, and work through any lingering effects of the toxic relationship.

Seeking support after getting out of a toxic relationship is crucial for healing, validation, and rebuilding your life. It provides a safe space to express your feelings and concerns, gain clarity, and receive guidance. Support from trusted individuals validates your experiences and offers reassurance that you made the right decision to leave. In addition, seeking professional help, such as therapy, can provide specialized guidance, coping strategies, and tools to navigate the healing process effectively. Remember, reaching out for support is a sign of strength and self-care, and it can be instrument-tal in your journey toward healing and creating healthier relationships.

Reach out to friends, family, or a therapist during this challenging time.

Reaching out to friends, family, or a therapist during this difficult time after getting out of a toxic relationship is essential for emotional support, validation, and professional guidance. Going through an unhealthy relationship can be emotionally draining and isolating, making connecting with others who can provide comfort and understanding crucial.

Friends and family members who are supportive can offer a listening ear and a safe space for you to share your experiences. They can provide emotional support, empathy, and validation, vital for healing and rebuilding your self-esteem. Trusted loved ones can help you see the toxic relationship from an outside perspective, offering insights and guidance that may be difficult to see on your own. Their presence and support can also remind you that you are not alone and that you have a support system to lean on.

In addition to friends and family, seeking the help of a therapist or counselor can be highly beneficial during this challenging time. A therapist is a trained professional who can provide objective guidance, strategies, and tools to help you navigate the healing process. They can help you process the toxic relationship's emotions, trauma, and impact in a safe and confidential environment. Therapists can assist in identifying patterns, healing from past wounds, rebuilding self-esteem, and developing healthy coping mechanisms. Their expertise can provide the professional guidance and support needed to heal and move forward healthily.

Reaching out to friends, family, or a therapist during this challenging time after getting out of a toxic relationship is essential for emotional support, validation, and professional guidance. Trusted loved ones can offer empathy, understanding, and an outside perspective, helping you navigate the healing process. Likewise, seeking the help of a therapist provides you with professional guidance, strategies, and tools to heal from the trauma and rebuild your life. Remember, reaching out for support is a courageous and important step toward your healing and personal growth.

Forgive yourself.

Forgiving yourself after getting out of a toxic relationship is essential for your emotional healing, self-compassion, and personal growth. Toxic relationships can often leave you feeling guilty, ashamed, or responsible for the dynamics and abuse that occurred. However, it is crucial to recognize that you were a victim of the toxic relationship and not to blame yourself for the other person's actions.

Forgiving yourself allows you to let go of self-blame and take back your power. It is essential to understand that you made the best decisions you could at the time, given the circumstances and the manipulation you may have experienced. By forgiving yourself, you release guilt and allow yourself to move forward with a renewed sense of self-worth.

Self-forgiveness also opens the door to self-compassion and self-care. It involves treating yourself with kindness, understanding, and acceptance. Recognizing that you deserve love, respect, and happiness helps you rebuild your self-esteem and trust. It allows you to focus on your well-being and prioritize your needs.

Furthermore, forgiving yourself promotes personal growth and resilience. It allows you to learn from experience and make positive changes in your life. By acknowledging the lessons learned from the toxic relationship, you can set healthier boundaries, develop more vital self-awareness, and establish new relationship patterns. Forgiving yourself creates space for personal growth and empowers you to create a more fulfilling and healthy future.

Forgiving yourself after getting out of a toxic relationship is essential for emotional healing, self-compassion, and personal growth. It allows you to let go of self-blame and reclaim your power. Forgiveness opens the door for self-compassion and self-care, fostering a sense of self-worth and well-being. It also promotes personal growth, resilience, and the opportunity to create healthier relationships in the future. Remember, forgiving yourself is a powerful act of self-love and an important step towards moving forward and embracing a brighter and more fulfilling life.

Let go of any shame or guilt.

Letting go of any shame or guilt after getting out of a toxic relationship is essential for your emotional healing, self-esteem, and overall well-being. In unhealthy relationships, abusers often manipulate and control their partners, making them feel responsible for the toxicity and abuse. However, it is crucial to understand that the blame lies solely with the abuser, and you should not carry the weight of shame or guilt for their actions.

Releasing shame and guilt allows you to reclaim your self-worth and break free from the cycle of self-blame. Please recognize that you were a victim of abuse and manipulation; it was not your fault. Acknowledge that the abuser's actions were a reflection of their issues and not a reflection of their worth or character. By letting go of shame and guilt, you create space for self-compassion, self-acceptance, and self-love.

Letting go of shame and guilt also empowers you to embrace personal growth and resilience. It enables you to focus on healing and moving forward rather than being stuck in the past. By releasing these negative emotions, you can free yourself from the constraints of the toxic relationship and open yourself up to new opportunities and healthier relationships. Embrace the lessons learned from the experience and use them as catalysts for personal growth, setting boundaries, and establishing healthier relationship dynamics in the future.

12 Steps to Recovering from A Toxic Relationship

Letting go of shame or guilt after getting out of a toxic relationship is vital for your emotional well-being and self-esteem. Understand that the blame lies solely with the abuser, and you are not responsible for their actions. Releasing shame and guilt allows you to reclaim your self-worth, practice self-compassion, and foster personal growth. By letting go of these negative emotions, you empower yourself to heal, move forward, and create a brighter future filled with self-love and healthier relationships. Remember, you deserve to let go of any shame or guilt and embrace a life of happiness and emotional freedom.

Practice self-compassion.

Practicing self-compassion after exiting a toxic relationship is essential for healing, self-esteem, and overall well-being. Toxic relationships can leave deep emotional wounds and often lead to feelings of self-blame, inadequacy, and worthlessness. However, by cultivating self-compassion, you can offer the same kindness, understanding, and support you would extend to a loved one in a similar situation.

Self-compassion involves treating yourself with warmth, empathy, and acceptance. It means acknowledging the pain and suffering you experienced in the toxic relationship without judgment. By recognizing that you were a victim of abuse and manipulation, you can shift the blame away from yourself and begin to heal from the emotional scars. In addition, embracing self-compassion allows you to validate your feelings and experiences, creating a safe space for healing and self-growth.

Moreover, self-compassion helps to rebuild your self-esteem and sense of self-worth. By practicing self-compassion, you can challenge the negative beliefs and self-critical thoughts that may have been instilled during the toxic relationship. Instead, you learn to reframe your experiences with kindness and understanding, realizing that your worth and value are not determined by the toxic dynamics you endured. This shift in perspective empowers you to rebuild your self-esteem and develop a healthier and more positive relationship with yourself.

Practicing self-compassion also sets the foundation for establishing healthier boundaries and engaging in self-care. It involves prioritizing your well-being, recognizing your needs, and honoring them without guilt. Self-compassion allows you to nurture yourself physically and emotionally and create a supportive environment that promotes healing and growth. By showing yourself compassion, you open the door to personal transformation, resilience, and the ability to cultivate healthier relationships in the future.

Practicing self-compassion after exiting a toxic relationship is vital for your emotional healing, self-esteem, and personal growth. It involves treating yourself with kindness, empathy, and acceptance, acknowledging that you were a victim of abuse and manipulation. Self-compassion helps to rebuild your self-worth, challenge negative beliefs, and establish healthier boundaries. By embracing self-compassion, you create a foundation for healing, self-care, and navigating future relationships with greater self-love and compassion. Remember, you deserve to treat yourself with the same care and understanding that you would extend to others in need.

<u>Engage in positive activities.</u>

Engaging in positive activities after getting out of a toxic relationship is essential for healing, personal growth, and overall well-being. Toxic relationships can leave you emotionally drained, depleted, and with a negative outlook on life. Conversely, you can restore a sense of joy, purpose, and fulfillment by actively seeking out and participating in positive activities.

Positive activities distract from the pain and negative emotions associated with the toxic relationship. They allow you to shift your focus toward activities that bring you happiness, peace, and a sense of accomplishment. Engaging in hobbies, exercise, creative outlets, or spending time in nature can help you reconnect with yourself and rediscover your passions and interests. You create space for healing and personal growth by immersing yourself in positive activities.

Furthermore, positive activities promote self-care and self-nurturing. After a toxic relationship, it is crucial to prioritize your well-being and reestablish a positive relationship with yourself. Engaging in activities that bring you joy, relaxation, or a sense of achievement allows you to nurture your physical, emotional, and mental health. By investing time and energy into positive activities, you reaffirm your self-worth and reinforce the importance of self-care in your life.

Participating in positive activities also helps in rebuilding your self-esteem and confidence. Toxic relationships often erode your sense of self and make you doubt your abilities and worthiness. Engaging in positive activities provides opportunities to challenge those negative beliefs and prove to yourself that you are capable, talented, and deserving of happiness. As you accomplish small goals or enjoy these activities, you strengthen your self-esteem and gain confidence in your abilities.

Engaging in positive activities after getting out of a toxic relationship is essential for healing, personal growth, and overall well-being. By participating in activities that bring you joy, purpose, and a sense of accomplishment, you can shift your focus towards positivity and create space for healing. Positive activities are a form of self-care and self-nurturing, allowing you to prioritize your well-being. They also help rebuild your self-esteem and confidence as you prove you can achieve happiness and success. Remember, engaging in positive activities is a powerful tool for post-toxic relationship recovery and can contribute to a brighter and more fulfilling future. Be patient and trust the process: Healing from a toxic relationship can be a long and challenging journey, but trusting and being patient with yourself is essential. Remember that you are strong and capable of overcoming this difficult time. Healing takes time, and trusting and being patient with yourself are crucial. By

12 Steps to Recovering from A Toxic Relationship

offering yourself patience and grace, you can move forward and create a healthier and happier life. Preventing yourself from blaming yourself for your part in a toxic relationship requires recognizing that toxicity in a relationship is often a result of a pattern of behavior between two people, not just one person's actions. Acknowledging your role in the relationship is essential, but it is equally important to recognize that you are not solely responsible for the toxicity. Practice self-compassion and remind yourself that your past experiences do not define you. Seek support from friends, family, or a therapist who can help you process your emotions and offer a different perspective. By stepping back and focusing on personal growth and healing, you can work towards forgiving yourself and letting go of any self-blame, ultimately creating a positive and healthy future for yourself.

Step 5. Face Your Pain, Don't Be Scare To Accept Your Discomfort

After getting out of a toxic relationship, it's common to feel pain and discomfort as you work through your emotions and begin healing. However, facing your pain and accepting your discomfort is essential rather than trying to push it away or ignore it. By acknowledging your pain and allowing yourself to feel it, you can begin to process your emotions and work towards healing. Seek support from friends, family, or a therapist, and practice self-care activities such as exercise, meditation, or therapy. It's important to be patient with yourself and understand that healing takes time. Identify your triggers and take steps to avoid them when possible.

Acknowledge your pain.

Acknowledging your pain after getting out of a toxic relationship is essential for your healing, growth, and overall well-being. Unhealthy relationships often inflict deep emotional wounds, leaving you feeling broken, hurt, and confused. Acknowledging and validating your pain allows you to begin healing and moving forward.

Acknowledging your pain is an important step towards understanding the impact of the toxic relationship on your life. It involves allowing yourself to feel and express your emotions without judgment or shame. By acknowledging the pain, you can start unraveling the complex layers of hurt, betrayal, and manipulation you may have experienced. In addition, this self-awareness allows you to make sense of your emotions, thoughts, and reactions and helps you regain control over your narrative.

Furthermore, acknowledging your pain creates space for healing and growth. It enables you to confront and process the emotions that may have been suppressed or ignored during the toxic relationship. By permitting yourself to feel the pain, you open the door to healing and release. This process may involve seeking support from therapists, support groups, or trusted friends and family who can provide a safe space to express your feelings and offer guidance on navigating the healing journey.

Acknowledging your pain also paves the way for self-compassion and self-forgiveness. By recognizing the depth of your pain, you can extend compassion and understanding to yourself, realizing that you are not to blame for the toxic dynamics of the relationship. Acknowledging your pain allows you to release any self-judgment or guilt that may have been weighing you down and instead focus on your healing and growth. This self-compassion provides a solid foundation for rebuilding your self-esteem, reclaiming your power, and establishing healthier relationships in the future.

Acknowledging your pain after getting out of a toxic relationship is crucial for healing, growth, and overall well-being. By accepting your pain, you allow yourself to understand and process the impact of the toxic relationship and make sense of your emotions and reactions. This self-awareness creates space for healing, growth, and releasing suppressed emotions. Acknowledging your pain also enables you to practice self-compassion and self-forgiveness and rebuild your self-esteem. Remember, owning your pain is a courageous step towards reclaiming your happiness, self-worth and creating a brighter future.

Be kind to yourself.

Being kind to yourself after getting out of a toxic relationship is essential for your healing, self-esteem, and overall well-being. Toxic relationships can leave you feeling depleted, insecure, and unworthy of love and kindness. By intentionally practicing self-kindness, you can counteract the adverse effects of the toxic relationship and rebuild a positive relationship with yourself.

Being kind to yourself involves treating yourself with compassion, understanding, and forgiveness. It means acknowledging that you deserve love, respect, and care, regardless of the toxic dynamics you endured. By extending kindness to yourself, you shift the narrative from self-blame and self-criticism to self-acceptance and self-empowerment.

Practicing self-kindness also helps to rebuild your self-esteem. Toxic relationships often chip away at your confidence and make you question your worth. By actively being kind to yourself, you challenge the negative beliefs and self-doubt that may have been instilled during the toxic relationship. You embrace your inherent value and recognize that you deserve kindness, compassion, and respect. This shift in perspective allows you to rebuild your self-esteem and cultivate a healthier, more positive self-image.

Moreover, being kind to yourself promotes healing and personal growth. It creates a nurturing environment for your emotional well-being and provides space for self-reflection, self-care, and self-discovery. By practicing self-kindness, you prioritize your needs, set healthy boundaries, and engage in activities that bring you joy and fulfillment. It allows you to let go of the negativity from the past and focus on your present and future, fostering a sense of empowerment and resilience.

Being kind to yourself after getting out of a toxic relationship is essential for your healing, self-esteem, and personal growth. It involves treating yourself with compassion, understanding, and forgiveness. By practicing self-kindness, you counteract the adverse effects of the toxic relationship and rebuild a positive relationship with yourself. Being kind to yourself helps to restore self-esteem, challenge self-doubt, and cultivate self-acceptance. It also promotes healing and personal growth as you prioritize self-care and engage in activities that bring you joy and fulfillment. Remember, you deserve to be kind to yourself and create a life filled with love, compassion, and happiness.

Seek support,

Seeking support after getting out of a toxic relationship is essential for healing, recovery, and overall well-being. Toxic relationships can leave deep emotional wounds and often result in feelings of isolation, confusion, and self-doubt. By reaching out for support, you create a network of understanding individuals who can provide guidance, validation, and a safe space for you to heal and grow.

Seeking support allows you to break the cycle of silence and secrecy that often accompanies toxic relationships. It will enable you to share your experiences, feelings, and concerns with trusted friends, family members, or professionals who can offer a listening ear and empathetic support. By voicing your experiences, you validate your feelings and gain clarity about the dynamics of the toxic relationship. This external validation can be instrumental in rebuilding your self-esteem and regaining your sense of self.

Moreover, seeking support helps you to gain perspective and insight into the dynamics of the toxic relationship. Friends, family, or therapists can provide an outside perspective, helping you identify patterns, recognize red flags, and gain a deeper understanding of the dynamics that contributed to the toxicity. In addition, they can offer guidance, resources, and coping strategies to help you navigate the healing process and move forward healthily and empowered. Having a support system also serves as a reminder

12 Steps to Recovering from A Toxic Relationship

that you are not alone and that there are people who care about your well-being.

Additionally, seeking support fosters a sense of community and connection. Surrounding yourself with supportive individuals who understand and validate your experiences can be incredibly empowering. They can provide a sense of belonging and help you rebuild trust in others after the trauma of a toxic relationship. Together, you can share experiences, learn from one another, and support each other's healing journey. A community's collective strength and support can be instrumental in rebuilding your confidence, self-worth, and resilience.

Seeking support after getting out of a toxic relationship is essential for healing, recovery, and overall well-being. First, it breaks the cycle of silence and isolation, providing a safe space to share and process your experiences. Seeking support helps you gain perspective, insights, and coping strategies to navigate the healing process. Finally, it fosters a sense of community and connection, reminding you that you are not alone. Remember, reaching out for support is a courageous step towards reclaiming your happiness, healing, and building a supportive network of individuals who will empower and uplift you.

Keith L. Belvin

Practice self-care.

Practicing self-care is essential for dealing with the pain and trauma that can linger after getting out of a toxic relationship. Toxic relationships can leave you emotionally drained, with diminished self-esteem and struggling with negative emotions. By prioritizing self-care, you can nurture your physical, emotional, and mental well-being, promoting healing and restoring balance.

Self-care involves intentionally engaging in activities that promote self-nurturing and self-compassion. It means listening to your needs and prioritizing activities that bring you joy, relaxation, and a sense of peace. Practicing self-care sends a powerful message to yourself that you are worthy of love, care, and happiness. This self-validation can counteract the negative messages and experiences from the toxic relationship and help you rebuild your self-esteem.

Additionally, self-care serves as a coping mechanism and a way to manage the pain and emotional turmoil that may accompany the aftermath of a toxic relationship. Engaging in self-care activities such as exercise, meditation, journaling, or time in nature can help alleviate stress, reduce anxiety, and promote emotional healing. By investing time and energy into self-care, you create a safe space for yourself to process your emotions, release negativity, and cultivate a sense of inner peace.

Practicing self-care also supports your overall recovery and resilience. It allows you to replenish your energy, restore balance, and rebuild your emotional strength. In addition, self-care activities can provide a sense of empowerment and control over your well-being, reminding you that you have the power to nurture and heal yourself. As you consistently practice self-care, you cultivate a foundation of self-love, self-compassion, and self-empowerment that can be a strong pillar in your healing journey and moving forward.

Self-care is essential for dealing with the pain and trauma after getting out of a toxic relationship. It promotes healing, restores balance, and nurtures your overall well-being. By prioritizing self-care, you affirm your self-worth, rebuild your self-esteem, and send a message of self-love and self-compassion. Self-care is a coping mechanism allowing you to manage and process your emotions. It also supports your recovery and resilience, providing a foundation of strength and empowerment as you navigate your healing journey. Remember, practicing self-care is a powerful act of self-love and an investment in your well-being.

Identify your triggers.

Identifying your triggers is essential for dealing with the pain and emotional aftermath of getting out of a toxic relationship. Toxic relationships can leave deep emotional wounds and residual trauma that can resurface in certain situations or interactions. By becoming aware of your triggers, you gain insight into the specific circumstances or behaviors that evoke negative emotions, allowing you to develop effective strategies for managing and healing from them.

Identifying your triggers involves paying attention to your emotional and physical responses in various situations. It requires self-reflection and introspection to recognize patterns and associations between specific triggers and your emotional reactions. By understanding what triggers, you can better anticipate and prepare for them, making it easier to navigate and manage your emotional responses.

Once you have identified your triggers, you can implement healthy coping mechanisms and self-care strategies to address them. This may involve engaging in relaxation techniques, practicing mindfulness, seeking support from trusted individuals, or engaging in therapeutic activities such as journaling or therapy. By proactively managing your triggers, you regain control over your emotional well-being and create a safe space for healing and growth.

Moreover, identifying your triggers helps break the cycle of re-traumatization. Toxic relationships can create deeply ingrained patterns and beliefs that perpetuate negative emotions and behaviors. By recognizing your triggers, you can challenge and reframe these patterns, fostering a sense of empowerment and promoting positive change. By consciously addressing and healing from your triggers, you can break free from the emotional entanglement of the toxic relationship and create healthier, more fulfilling relationships in the future.

12 Steps to Recovering from A Toxic Relationship

Identifying your triggers is essential for dealing with a toxic relationship's pain and emotional aftermath. It allows you to gain insight into the specific circumstances or behaviors that evoke negative emotions, empowering you to develop effective strategies for managing and healing from them. By recognizing your triggers, you can implement healthy coping mechanisms and self-care strategies to address them, promoting emotional well-being and growth. Moreover, identifying your triggers helps break the cycle of re-traumatization and allows you to challenge and reframe negative patterns, creating a foundation for healthier relationships and personal transformation. Remember, identifying your triggers is a decisive step towards healing and reclaiming your emotional well-being.

<u>Let yourself grieve.</u>

Letting yourself grieve is essential for dealing with the pain and emotional turmoil that follows getting out of a toxic relationship. Toxic relationships can cause deep emotional wounds, leaving you with loss, betrayal, and heartbreak. Allowing yourself to grieve gives you permission to acknowledge and process these painful emotions, facilitating healing and paving the way for emotional growth. Grief is a natural response to loss, and the end of a toxic relationship signifies the loss of a dream, the loss of the person you thought they were, and the loss of the future you had envisioned. By allowing yourself to grieve, you honor the depth of your emotions and give yourself the space to mourn the loss of what could have been. This process will enable you to release pent-up emotions and begin the healing journey.

Letting yourself grieve also means validating your experiences and emotions. In a toxic relationship, you may have been gaslighted, manipulated, or made to doubt your reality. Grieving allows you to affirm your truth and acknowledge the pain you endured. By validating your experiences, you reclaim your power and rebuild your self-esteem, reminding yourself that your emotions are valid and deserve acknowledgment.

Moreover, the grieving process enables you to gain closure and move forward. By allowing yourself to feel and process the pain, you can gradually release the toxic relationship and its hold on your emotions. It provides an opportunity to reflect on the lessons learned, and the growth achieved, and the qualities you seek in healthy relationships. Grieving allows you to release the past and open yourself up to new possibilities and more beneficial connections.

Letting yourself grieve is essential for dealing with the pain after getting out of a toxic relationship. It honors the depth of your emotions, validates your experiences, and provides healing and growth opportunities. By allowing yourself to grieve, you release pent-up emotions, gain closure, and pave the way for a brighter future. Remember, grieving is a natural and necessary process that allows you to reclaim your emotional well-being and create space for healthier relationships in the future.

12 Steps to Recovering from A Toxic Relationship

Forgive yourself.

Forgiving yourself is essential for dealing with the pain and emotional aftermath of getting out of a toxic relationship. Toxic relationships often leave individuals with self-blame, guilt, and shame as they question their judgment or actions. However, forgiving yourself is a powerful act of self-compassion that can free you from self-blame and allow you to heal and move forward.

Forgiving yourself means acknowledging that you did the best you could with the knowledge and resources you had at the time. In a toxic relationship, you may have been manipulated, gaslighted, or made to feel responsible for the dysfunction. By forgiving yourself, you release the unrealistic expectations and self-judgment, recognizing that you were a victim of toxic dynamics. It is important to remember that you deserve compassion and understanding, just like anyone else.

Additionally, forgiving yourself helps you reclaim your power and self-worth. Toxic relationships often erode self-esteem and create a distorted self-image. By forgiving yourself, you acknowledge that you are not defined by the toxic relationship or the mistakes you made. It allows you to challenge negative beliefs and replace them with self-compassion and self-love. Forgiving yourself is a transformative process that lets you let go of the past and embrace your inherent worthiness.

Furthermore, forgiving yourself opens the door to personal growth and new possibilities. It frees up mental and emotional space previously occupied by self-blame and regret. By letting go of the pain and forgiving yourself, you create room for self-discovery, self-improvement, and the pursuit of healthier relationships. Forgiveness allows you to break free from the chains of the past and embrace a future filled with self-compassion, personal growth, and joy.

Forgiving yourself is essential for dealing with the pain after getting out of a toxic relationship. It involves releasing self-blame, guilt, and shame and embracing self-compassion and self-love. By forgiving yourself, you acknowledge that you did the best you could and free yourself from the burden of unrealistic expectations. It is a transformative process that allows you to reclaim your power and self-worth and create space for personal growth and healthier relationships. Remember, forgiveness is a gift you give yourself and an essential step in your healing journey.

Engage in positive activities.

Engaging in positive activities is essential for dealing with the pain and emotional aftermath of getting out of a toxic relationship. Toxic relationships can leave individuals feeling drained, depleted, and emotionally scarred. By intentionally incorporating positive activities into your life, you can shift your focus towards healing, self-care, and personal growth.

12 Steps to Recovering from A Toxic Relationship

Positive activities provide a much-needed respite from the pain and negativity associated with a toxic relationship. They distract from intrusive thoughts and painful memories, allowing you to redirect your energy toward activities that bring you joy, fulfillment, and a sense of well-being. Whether engaging in hobbies, pursuing creative outlets, practicing mindfulness, or spending time in nature, positive activities create space for positivity and help restore a sense of balance and inner peace.

Engaging in positive activities also promotes self-discovery and personal growth. Toxic relationships can leave individuals feeling lost, disconnected from their passions, and unsure of their identity. By immersing yourself in positive activities, you can reconnect with yourself, explore new interests, and rediscover your strengths and talents. These activities provide a platform for self-expression, self-reflection, and personal development, allowing you to rebuild your sense of self and establish a fulfilling and authentic life.

Moreover, positive activities foster a sense of empowerment and self-care. They remind you that you deserve happiness, pleasure, and self-indulgence. Engaging in activities that bring you joy and fulfillment can help rewire your brain to associate positivity and self-worth with your actions and choices. By prioritizing self-care and engaging in activities that nourish your mind, body, and soul, you send a powerful message to yourself that you are worthy of love, happiness, and a life free from toxicity.

Engaging in positive activities is essential for dealing with the pain after getting out of a toxic relationship. They provide a much-needed respite from negativity and distract from painful memories. In addition, positive activities promote self-discovery, personal growth, and empowerment, allowing you to reconnect with yourself and establish a fulfilling life. They also serve as a powerful tool for self-care and reinforce your self-worth and deservingness of happiness. Remember, engaging in positive activities is vital to healing, reclaiming your joy, and creating a life filled with positivity and fulfillment.

Be patient.

Being patient is essential for dealing with the pain and emotional healing after getting out of a toxic relationship. Recovering from the aftermath of a toxic relationship takes time, and it is crucial to be patient with yourself as you navigate the healing difficulties.

Firstly, it is essential to acknowledge that healing is not linear. There will be good and bad days, moments of progress, and setbacks. Being patient allows you to accept that healing takes time and that it is okay to have moments of vulnerability or to experience lingering pain. It is a process of untangling emotional complexities and rebuilding yourself, and being patient enables you to give yourself the necessary time and space to heal at your own pace.

Furthermore, being patient with yourself fosters self-compassion. In a toxic relationship, you may have internalized negative beliefs about yourself or been subjected to blame and criticism. By practicing patience, you counteract these damaging narratives and show yourself kindness and understanding. You acknowledge that healing is a journey and deserves patience and gentleness. This self-compassion is crucial for building resilience and nurturing your self-esteem.

Lastly, being patient allows you to honor the healing process and appreciate the progress you make along the way. Getting caught up in wanting to feel better quickly or comparing your healing timeline with others is easy. However, being patient shifts your focus from immediate relief to long-term growth. You recognize that healing is gradual and celebrate even the smallest steps forward. This perspective cultivates gratitude, resilience, and a deeper understanding of yourself.

Being patient is essential for dealing with the pain after getting out of a toxic relationship. It enables you to accept the non-linear nature of healing, foster self-compassion, and appreciate the progress you make. Being patient with yourself honors the healing journey, allowing for emotional growth and rebuilding your life. Remember, healing takes time, and by being patient, you provide yourself with the space and support necessary to emerge stronger, wiser, and ready for a healthier future.

Accept discomfort:

Accepting discomfort is essential for dealing with the pain and emotional challenges that arise after getting out of a toxic relationship. When you leave a toxic relationship, it is natural to experience a range of uncomfortable emotions such as sadness, anger, fear, and confusion. However, allowing yourself to accept and sit with these discomforts creates space for healing and growth.

Firstly, accepting discomfort allows you to validate your emotions. It is common to want to avoid or suppress painful feelings, as they can be overwhelming. However, by accepting discomfort, you acknowledge the validity of your emotions and permit yourself to experience them fully. This acceptance process is an important step towards healing, as it allows you to process and release pent-up emotions rather than burying them deep within.

Secondly, accepting discomfort helps you gain insight and self-awareness. When you allow yourself to sit with uncomfortable emotions, you create an opportunity for self-reflection and understanding. By examining your feelings and their underlying causes, you can identify patterns, triggers, and areas for personal growth. Through this self-reflection, you can heal old wounds, challenge limiting beliefs, and make positive changes in your life.

Lastly, accepting discomfort fosters resilience and personal growth. It takes courage to face and accept uncomfortable emotions head-on. However, by embracing pain, you develop resilience and inner strength. You learn to navigate complex emotions and situations with greater ease and self-assurance. This resilience enables you to grow and evolve from the pain, transforming it into wisdom, compassion, and a greater sense of self.

Accepting discomfort is essential for dealing with the pain after getting out of a toxic relationship. It allows you to validate your emotions, gain insight and self-awareness, and foster resilience and personal growth. In addition, accepting discomfort creates space for healing, self-reflection, and transformation. Remember, discomfort is a natural part of the healing process, and by taking it, you open the door to greater self-discovery, healing, and a brighter future. Let yourself grieve and forgive yourself for any mistakes you may have made in the relationship. Engage in positive activities and be kind to yourself as you navigate the healing process. Remember facing your pain and discomfort is a brave and necessary step toward healing and moving forward. Meeting one's pain and not being scared to accept hurt requires a willingness to sit with and process difficult emotions. It can be tempting to avoid pain or discomfort by distracting oneself with other activities or behaviors, but this can ultimately prolong the healing process. By allowing yourself to feel and process your emotions, you can begin to understand what happened and work towards healing and moving forward. It is vital to approach this process with self-compassion and patience, recognizing that healing is not a linear process and that it may take time. Seek support from loved ones or a therapist who can provide guidance and a safe space to explore your emotions. By facing your pain and discomfort head-on, you can work towards finding closure and ultimately create a positive future for yourself.

Step 6: Getting Closure Is On You, Not The Person Who Hurt You.

The idea of getting closure is on you, not the person who hurt you, suggests that finding peace and moving on from a situation lies within your control and not in the actions of others. It highlights the importance of taking responsibility for your emotional healing and recognizing that closure is a personal journey that requires self-reflection, self-care, and self-compassion. By accepting this idea, you empower yourself to let go of the past, focus on the present, and create a positive future for yourself, regardless of the actions of others.

Acknowledge your feelings.

Acknowledging your feelings is essential for obtaining closure after getting out of a toxic relationship. When you exit a toxic relationship, you may experience a whirlwind of emotions such as anger, sadness, confusion, or relief. Acknowledging and validating these feelings to process them effectively and ultimately find closure is crucial.

Firstly, acknowledging your feelings allows you to honor your emotional experience. Denying or suppressing your emotions can prolong the healing process and hinder closure. By recognizing and accepting your feelings, you give yourself permission to experience and express them authentically. This validation is essential to healing as it helps you reclaim your emotional agency and regain control over your well-being.

Secondly, acknowledging your feelings enables you to gain clarity and understanding. Emotions serve as valuable signals that provide insight into your experiences and needs. By acknowledging your feelings, you create an opportunity for self-reflection and introspection. It allows you to identify patterns, recognize unhealthy dynamics, and understand the toxic relationship's impact on you. This newfound understanding empowers you to make informed decisions and establish healthier boundaries in future relationships.

Lastly, acknowledging your feelings paves the way for closure and moving forward. Closure does not necessarily mean having all the answers or a tidy resolution. Instead, it means reaching a point where you have processed your emotions, accepted the reality of the situation, and are ready to let go. Acknowledging your feelings releases emotional baggage and creates space for healing and personal growth. It allows you to shift your focus towards rebuilding your life, cultivating self-love, and embracing new opportunities.

In conclusion, acknowledging your feelings is essential for obtaining closure after getting out of a toxic relationship. It allows you to honor your emotional experience, gain clarity and understanding, and pave the way for closure and moving forward. Remember, acknowledging your feelings is a powerful act of self-care and self-empowerment. Embracing your emotions lays the foundation for healing, resilience, and a future filled with healthier and more fulfilling relationships.

Accept that closure is a process:

Getting closure after getting out of a toxic relationship can be challenging and emotional. One helpful approach is to accept that closure is a process rather than an instantaneous event. By understanding this, you can give yourself the time and space needed to heal and move forward.

Firstly, it is essential to acknowledge that closure cannot be achieved overnight. Healing from the wounds inflicted by a toxic relationship takes time and patience. It is a multifaceted process involving various emotions, such as anger, sadness, and betrayal. Recognize that there will be good and bad days and that it is natural to experience setbacks. Embrace that healing is not linear but a series of difficulties. By accepting this, you can permit yourself to grieve and process your emotions at your own pace. Secondly, understand that closure doesn't necessarily come from external factors or actions from your ex-partner. While seeking closure from them is common, it is crucial to recognize that closure ultimately comes from within yourself. It's about finding inner peace and understanding that you are not defined by your ex-partner's toxic relationship or actions. Focus on self-reflection and personal growth. Engage in self-care activities that help you rebuild and regain your self-esteem. Surround yourself with a supportive network of friends and loved ones who can provide guidance and encouragement during this challenging time.

Lastly, be compassionate with yourself throughout the closure process. Understand that healing takes time and that it's okay to have setbacks or moments of vulnerability—practice self-compassion by being patient and gentle with yourself. Allow yourself to feel the emotions that arise without judgment or self-criticism. Remember that healing is a journey, and it's essential to celebrate even the most minor steps forward. By accepting that closure is a process, you can release the pressure to achieve immediate closure and instead focus on your personal growth and well-being.

In summary, accepting that closure is a process allows you to approach healing from a toxic relationship with patience, self-compassion, and a realistic outlook. First, give yourself the time and space to heal, understanding that it's a journey with ups and downs. Next, recognize that closure comes from within and focus on self-reflection and personal growth. Finally, be kind to yourself throughout the process, embracing each step forward and practicing self-compassion. With these approaches, you can gain closure and move toward a healthier and happier future.

12 Steps to Recovering from A Toxic Relationship

Recognize that closure comes from within.

Recognizing that closure comes from within is a powerful way to gain closure after getting out of a toxic relationship. Firstly, it's essential to understand that seeking external validation or closure from the toxic partner may not be productive or even possible. Waiting for them to apologize or provide the closure you seek can lead to prolonged pain and frustration. Instead, shifting the focus inward allows you to take control of your healing process. By acknowledging that closure is a personal journey, you empower yourself to find the resolution and peace you need within yourself.

Secondly, recognizing that closure comes from within enables you to explore your emotions, needs, and boundaries. Rather than relying on the toxic partner for validation or closure, you can turn inward and reflect on your own experiences and reactions. Take the time to process your emotions, whether it's through therapy, journaling, or talking to trusted friends or family members. By understanding and honoring your feelings, you can begin to make sense of the relationship dynamics and their impact on you. This self-awareness and self-reflection are crucial for healing and finding the necessary closure.

Lastly, recognizing that closure comes from within allows you to redefine your narrative and regain power. Toxic relationships can leave us feeling disempowered and questioning our self-worth. By understanding that closure is not about the toxic partner's actions or lack thereof but about finding peace and acceptance within yourself, you reclaim your sense of agency. You can redefine your story, separate your identity from the relationship's toxicity, and focus on personal growth and happiness. This recognition empowers you to move forward, heal, and create a brighter future for yourself, independent of the toxic influences of the past.

In summary, recognizing that closure comes from within is a transformative way to gain closure after leaving a toxic relationship. It lets you let go of the need for external validation, explore your emotions and conditions, and redefine your narrative. By shifting the focus inward, you take control of your healing process and empower yourself to find resolution, peace, and acceptance within yourself. Remember, closure is a personal journey, and by recognizing this, you can move forward, heal, and create a life free from the toxic influences of the past.

Reframe the situation.

Reframing the situation is a powerful way to gain closure after getting out of a toxic relationship. Firstly, it's important to shift your perspective and reframe the narrative of the relationship. Instead of viewing yourself as a victim or blaming yourself for the toxicity, recognize that you had the strength and courage to leave the toxic situation. Next, reframe the experience as a learning opportunity where you gain valuable insights about your boundaries, needs, and the qualities you desire in a healthy relationship. Finally, by reframing the situation as a catalyst for personal growth, you can let go of self-blame and embrace a more empowering perspective.

Secondly, reframe the meaning you attach to the relationship and the breakup. Rather than viewing it as a failure or a reflection of your worth, consider it a steppingstone towards a healthier and more fulfilling future. Recognize that the toxic relationship served as a valuable lesson in identifying red flags, setting boundaries, and prioritizing your well-being. Reframing the breakup as a necessary and positive step toward personal growth allows you to detach yourself from lingering negative emotions and gain closure. Embrace the idea that the end of the toxic relationship opens up new possibilities and paves the way for healthier connections in the future.

Lastly, reframe your focus on self-care and self-love. Use the closure process to prioritize your well-being and nurture yourself. Engage in activities that bring you joy, practice self-compassion, and surround yourself with supportive people. Reframe your energy towards healing and personal growth, investing in your happiness and fulfillment. By shifting the focus from the toxic relationship to self-care, you reclaim your power and create a positive and nurturing environment for closure. This reframing allows you to let go of the toxic past and create a brighter future built on self-love and resilience.

In summary, reframing the situation is a powerful tool to gain closure after leaving a toxic relationship. You can find peace and closure by shifting your perspective, reframing the narrative, and redirecting your focus toward personal growth and self-care. Embrace the lessons learned, view the breakup as necessary for a healthier future, and prioritize your well-being. Reframing allows you to let go of the negative emotions and experiences associated with the toxic relationship and create a positive foundation for closure and personal transformation.

Forgive yourself.

Forgiving yourself is crucial in gaining closure after getting out of a toxic relationship. Firstly, it's essential to acknowledge that it's normal to feel guilt, shame, or self-blame after leaving a toxic relationship. However, holding onto these negative emotions only prolongs the healing process. To forgive yourself, start by recognizing that you made the best decision you could at the time, given the circumstances and the information available. Next, understand that you are not responsible for the toxic behavior of your partner and that you deserve love, respect, and a healthy relationship. Finally, by shifting the blame from yourself to the toxic dynamics of the relationship, you can begin to let go of self-judgment and move toward forgiveness.

Secondly, practice self-compassion and kindness towards yourself. Understand that you are human and that everyone makes mistakes. Treat yourself with the same understanding and compassion you would offer

12 Steps to Recovering from A Toxic Relationship

a close friend in a similar situation. Acknowledge the pain you experienced in the toxic relationship, and instead of criticizing yourself for staying or for any perceived shortcomings, offer yourself love and empathy. Embrace that you took the brave step of leaving the toxic relationship and forgive yourself for any perceived missteps. Self-forgiveness allows you to release the burden of self-blame and creates space for healing and closure.

Lastly, focus on personal growth and self-improvement. Use the lessons learned from the toxic relationship as an opportunity for self-reflection and growth. Identify areas where you can strengthen your boundaries, enhance your self-esteem, and develop healthier relationship patterns. By committing to your growth and development, you demonstrate that you have learned from the experience and are actively working towards a better future. In addition, this dedication to personal growth and improvement helps foster forgiveness towards yourself as you recognize that you are taking the necessary steps to heal and move forward.

In summary, forgiving yourself is essential to gaining closure after leaving a toxic relationship. Recognize that you made the best decisions you could at the time and that you are not to blame for the toxic behavior of your partner. Practice self-compassion and treat yourself with kindness, acknowledging that you are human and deserving of love and respect. Focus on personal growth and improvement, using the lessons learned to enhance your boundaries and develop healthier relationship patterns. By forgiving yourself, you release the burden of self-blame and create space for healing, closure, and a brighter future.

Create closure rituals:

Creating closure rituals can be a meaningful and cathartic way to gain closure after getting out of a toxic relationship. Firstly, consider the power of writing a closure letter to your toxic partner. This letter should express your emotions, thoughts, and experiences, allowing you to release any pent-up feelings and gain a sense of closure. You can either keep the letter for your reflection or burn it as a symbolic act of letting go and freeing yourself from the emotional baggage of the toxic relationship. This ritual helps you externalize your emotions and start moving forward.

Secondly, consider creating a physical representation of closure through a symbolic object. For example, you can gather items that remind you of the toxic relationship and make a small ceremonial space. Take the time to reflect on each item and the associated emotions it brings up. Once you have acknowledged their significance, choose to let go of these items by disposing of them meaningfully. It could be burying them, throwing them into the water, or donating them to charity. By physically releasing these objects, you symbolically release the toxic energy they carry, allowing for closure and a fresh start.

12 Steps to Recovering from A Toxic Relationship

Lastly, consider engaging in a ritual of self-empowerment and affirmation. First, write down empowering statements or claims that counteract the negative beliefs or experiences from the toxic relationship. Then, stand before a mirror and recite these affirmations, allowing their positive energy to sink in and reshape your self-perception. Additionally, you can engage in a self-care activity that makes you feel strong and confident, such as taking a soothing bath, practicing yoga or meditation, or engaging in a favorite hobby. This ritual reinforces the idea that you deserve love, respect, and a healthy relationship, helping you to reclaim your power and create closure.

In summary, creating closure rituals can be a powerful tool for gaining closure after leaving a toxic relationship. Writing a closure letter and either keeping it or symbolically releasing it through burning can help externalize emotions and let go. Creating a symbolic object ceremony allows you to reflect on the significance of items from the toxic relationship and dispose of them, symbolizing the release of negative energy. Engaging in a ritual of self-empowerment and affirmation reinforces positive self-perception and self-care, facilitating closure and personal growth. These closure rituals provide a tangible and intentional way to mark the end of the toxic relationship and embark on a journey of healing and new beginnings.

Focus on the present.

Focusing on the present is a powerful way to gain closure after getting out of a toxic relationship. Firstly, practicing mindfulness and bringing your attention to the present moment is important. Next, acknowledge that the past is over and cannot be changed. By redirecting your focus to the present, you can shift your energy towards healing, self-discovery, and creating a positive future for yourself. Finally, embrace the present opportunities and consciously engage fully in the present moment through activities, relationships, or self-care practices. By living in the present, you break free from the grip of the toxic relationship and open yourself up to new experiences and possibilities.

Secondly, focus on self-reflection and personal growth. Use the lessons learned from the toxic relationship to catalyze self-discovery and self-improvement. Take the time to understand your own needs, values, and desires. Engage in activities that promote personal growth, such as therapy, journaling, or self-help workshops. By focusing on your growth and development, you empower yourself to create a future that aligns with your authentic self. Let go of the past and use it as a steppingstone to evolve into a more robust, wiser, and more resilient version of yourself. By staying present and committed to personal growth, you gain closure by moving forward in a positive direction.

Lastly, cultivate gratitude for the present moment. Shift your attention to what you are grateful for in your life. Practice gratitude exercises, such as keeping a journal or verbally expressing gratitude daily. By acknowledging the positive aspects of your life, you shift your focus away from the toxicity of the past and cultivate a sense of contentment and fulfillment in the present. Gratitude helps reframe your perspective, reminding you of the abundance and joy beyond the toxic relationship. By focusing on the present and embracing gratitude, you gain closure by fostering a positive mindset and nurturing a sense of fulfillment and happiness.

In summary, focusing on the present is a transformative way to recover after leaving a toxic relationship. First, practice mindfulness to shift your attention away from the past and embrace the present opportunities. Engage in self-reflection and personal growth to learn from the past and create a positive future. Finally, cultivate gratitude to foster a sense of contentment and fulfillment in the present. By staying present, committed to personal growth, and embracing gratitude, you gain closure by creating a life free from the toxicity of the past and filled with hope, joy, and personal fulfillment.

Practice self-care.

Practicing self-care is crucial to gaining closure after getting out of a toxic relationship. Firstly, prioritize your physical well-being by engaging in activities that promote your overall health. This can include regular exercise, eating nutritious meals, and getting enough sleep. Physical self-care benefits your physical health and contributes to your emotional well-being. When you care for your body, you message yourself that you are worthy of love, respect, and attention. Physical self-care can help restore your energy levels, boost your mood, and enhance your overall well-being, all essential to closure.

Secondly, focus on your emotional well-being by engaging in activities that nurture your mental and emotional health. This can involve engaging in therapeutic practices such as journaling, meditation, or seeking professional therapy. Finally, reflect on your emotions and allow yourself to process the feelings that arise from the toxic relationship. Give yourself permission to grieve, heal, and release any emotional baggage. By dedicating time to your emotional well-being, you create a safe space for healing and gain a deeper understanding of yourself and your needs. This self-reflection and emotional self-care are crucial in gaining closure as they allow you to acknowledge and work through the emotional impact of the toxic relationship.

Lastly, embrace activities that bring you joy, relaxation, and a sense of fulfillment. Engage in hobbies or creative outlets you enjoy, whether painting, playing an instrument, gardening, or dancing. Dedicate time to do what makes you feel alive and connected to your authentic self. Surround yourself with positive and supportive people who uplift and encourage you. Social self-care is vital in gaining closure as it helps build a support system and create new positive connections. By engaging in activities that bring you joy and surrounding yourself with positive influences, you reinforce your worthiness of happiness and fulfillment and create a nurturing environment for closure and personal growth.

Practicing self-care is a powerful way to gain closure after leaving a toxic relationship. Prioritize your physical well-being, engage in activities that promote emotional well-being, and embrace actions that bring you joy and fulfillment. Taking care of yourself conveys that you deserve love, respect, and attention. Engaging in self-care activities helps restore your energy, process emotions, and create a positive and nurturing environment for closure and personal growth. By prioritizing self-care, you empower yourself to heal, let go of the toxic past, and create a future filled with self-love, resilience, and happiness.

Seek professional help if needed.

Seeking professional help can be a valuable and necessary step in gaining closure after getting out of a toxic relationship. Firstly, suppose you find yourself unable to cope with the emotional aftermath of the toxic relationship, such as persistent feelings of sadness, anxiety, or anger. In that case, consulting a therapist or counselor may be beneficial. These professionals are trained to provide guidance and support tailored to your needs. They can help you navigate the complex emotions, trauma, and healing process of leaving a toxic relationship. They can also assist you in developing healthy coping mechanisms, processing your experiences, and rebuilding your self-esteem.

Secondly, notice significant disruptions in your daily functioning, such as difficulty concentrating at work or school, changes in appetite or sleep patterns, or a loss of interest in activities you once enjoyed. It may be a sign that professional help is needed. These disruptions may indicate underlying mental health concerns such as depression, anxiety, or post-traumatic stress disorder (PTSD) that require professional intervention. A therapist or psychiatrist can assess your symptoms and provide the appropriate diagnosis and treatment plan to support your healing journey. In addition, seeking professional help can offer you the tools and strategies needed to address these challenges effectively and regain a sense of stability and well-being.

Lastly, if you have experienced any form of abuse, whether it's physical, emotional, or sexual, it is crucial to seek professional help. Abuse can have long-lasting effects on your mental and emotional well-being, often requiring specialized support to navigate the healing process. Professionals specializing in trauma-informed care can help you address the specific challenges associated with abuse, providing a safe and supportive space to process your experiences, heal from the trauma, and regain a sense of safety and empowerment.

In summary, seeking professional help is important if you find yourself unable to cope with the emotional aftermath of a toxic relationship, experiencing disruptions in your daily functioning, or if you have experienced any form of abuse. Therapists, counselors, and other mental health professionals can provide tailored guidance, support, and treatment to help you navigate the healing process effectively. In addition, they can assist you in processing your emotions, developing healthy coping mechanisms, and rebuilding your sense of self. Remember, seeking professional help is not a sign of weakness but a courageous step towards healing, closure, and reclaiming your life after a toxic relationship.

Celebrate your progress.

Celebrating your progress is vital in gaining closure after getting out of a toxic relationship. Firstly, reflect on how far you have come since leaving the toxic relationship. Next, acknowledge your steps towards healing, personal growth, and creating a healthier life. Next, celebrate the moments of strength, resilience, and courage that have brought you to where you are today. Listing your big and small achievements and taking pride in each milestone can be helpful. Recognizing and celebrating your progress reinforces your ability to overcome adversity and build a positive future.

Secondly, create a ritual or special occasion to mark your progress and honor your journey. This could involve gathering with close friends or family members who have supported you throughout your healing process. Share your experiences, express your gratitude, and celebrate your resilience together. You can also consider treating yourself to a special outing or activity that brings you joy and a sense of accomplishment. It could be a spa day, a solo trip, or indulging in a favorite hobby or interest. By intentionally creating moments of celebration, you reinforce the significance of your progress and nurture a positive outlook on your journey toward closure.

Lastly, practice self-compassion and acknowledge that progress is not always linear. Healing from a toxic relationship is complex, and setbacks or challenging moments may occur. Instead of being discouraged by these moments, celebrate your resilience in getting back on track and continuing your journey toward closure. Offer yourself kindness, understanding, and patience during challenging times. Recognize that setbacks are opportunities for growth and learning and that every step forward is worth celebrating. By cultivating self-compassion and celebrating your resilience, you create a positive and supportive mindset that propels you toward closure and a brighter future.

In summary, celebrating your progress is essential in gaining closure after leaving a toxic relationship. Reflect on how far you have come, acknowledging your achievements and moments of strength. Create rituals or special occasions to honor your progress and share your journey with supportive loved ones. Treat yourself to special outings or activities that bring you joy and a sense of accomplishment. Practice self-compassion and celebrate your resilience, even in the face of setbacks. Celebrating your progress reinforces your ability to heal, grow, and create a positive future beyond the toxic relationship. Overall, these are excellent steps for accepting that getting closure is on you, not the person who hurt you. The only suggestion that may need improvement is creating closure rituals, which could be more specific on which types of ways to consider.

***Closure Rituals: ***

A closure ritual is a symbolic action or ceremony that marks the end of a chapter in your life and helps you move forward. It can be anything meaningful to you and enables you to symbolize the completion of a particular phase, such as a breakup, a job loss, or the end of a friendship. Closure rituals can be done alone or with others and can be simple or elaborate, depending on your preferences and the situation. Some examples of closure rituals include writing a letter to yourself or the person who hurt you and burning it, creating a vision board that represents your future goals and aspirations, or burying an object that represents the past. Closure rituals can be empowering and healing, allowing you to take control of the situation and find closure on your terms. By participating in a closure ritual, you acknowledge the ending of one chapter in your life and embrace the beginning of a new one.

Step 7: How To Keep Supportive People Around You After Getting Out Of Toxic Relationship

To Keep supportive people around you after getting out of a toxic relationship requires intentional effort and communication. It's important to identify the people in your life who have been there for you and who you trust to support you. Reach out to them and let them know you are going through a tough time, and we would appreciate their support. Communicate your needs clearly and be honest about what you are comfortable with. Be available for these relationships and show your appreciation for their help. It's also important to practice self-care and set boundaries, if necessary, to maintain healthy relationships. By prioritizing these relationships and intentionally keeping supportive people around you, you can create a robust support system and facilitate your healing process.

Identify your support system:

After getting out of a toxic relationship, identifying your support system and keeping supportive people around you is crucial. Firstly, take the time to assess the people in your life who have been consistently supportive, understanding, and empathetic. These individuals may be close friends, family members, or even support groups or therapists who have provided a safe space for you to share your experiences and emotions.

12 Steps to Recovering from A Toxic Relationship

Recognize the value these individuals bring to your life and their positive impact on your healing process. Then, communicate with them openly about your needs and the support you require, as they can offer valuable guidance, validation, and encouragement.

Secondly, it's crucial to establish clear boundaries with toxic or unsupportive individuals. Identify individuals who may have enabled or contributed to the toxic relationship and evaluate whether they are healthy to keep in your life moving forward. Limiting or cutting off contact with toxic people who hinder your progress and well-being may be necessary. Surrounding yourself with individuals who uplift and empower you is essential for gaining closure and building a healthier support system. Focus on cultivating relationships with people who genuinely care about your well-being, respect your boundaries, and support your growth.

Lastly, consider joining support groups or seeking professional help. Support groups provide a unique opportunity to connect with individuals who have experienced similar situations. They can offer empathy, understanding, and practical advice on navigating the challenges of healing from a toxic relationship. Therapy or counseling can also provide a safe and confidential space to process your emotions and receive guidance from a trained professional. These resources can be instrumental in helping you build a strong support system and gain closure after a toxic relationship.

In summary, identifying your support system and keeping supportive people around you after leaving a toxic relationship is vital. Assess the individuals who have consistently supported you and communicate openly with them about your needs. Establish boundaries with toxic individuals and focus on cultivating relationships with those who uplift and empower you. Consider joining support groups or seeking professional help to enhance your support network. By surrounding yourself with supportive people, you create a nurturing environment for healing, growth, and closure after a toxic relationship.

Reach out to them.

Reaching out to your support system is crucial in keeping supportive people around you after getting out of a toxic relationship. Firstly, identify the individuals in your support system you feel comfortable contacting. These may be close friends, family members, mentors, or support groups. Next, consider the individuals who have demonstrated understanding, empathy, and a willingness to listen without judgment. They are likely to be the ones who can provide the support and guidance you need during this challenging time.

Secondly, be proactive in reaching out to your support system. It can be challenging to ask for help, especially after going through a toxic relationship where you may have felt isolated or manipulated. However, remember that true friends and supportive individuals will be there

12 Steps to Recovering from A Toxic Relationship

for you when needed. Reach out to them and let them know what you're going through. Share your feelings, experiences, and concerns. Be open and honest about your need for support and ask for their assistance. By taking this step, you allow others to show up for you and strengthen the bonds within your support system.

Lastly, communicate your ongoing needs to your support system. Understand that healing from a toxic relationship is a process, and your needs may change over time. Keep the lines of communication open and update your support system about what you require from them. It could be a listening ear, advice, encouragement, or someone to spend time with. By expressing your needs, you ensure your support system remains responsive and attuned to your evolving healing journey. This open communication fosters trust, understanding, and a continued sense of support.

In summary, reaching out to your support system is essential in keeping supportive people around you after leaving a toxic relationship. Identify those who have demonstrated understanding and empathy. Be proactive in contacting them, sharing your experiences, and asking for support. Communicate your ongoing needs to ensure your support system remains responsive and understanding. By nurturing these relationships, you create a strong support network that can provide the care and encouragement you need to heal, gain closure, and move forward positively and healthily.

Be honest about your needs.

Being honest about your needs is crucial in keeping supportive people around you after getting out of a toxic relationship. Firstly, take the time to identify and understand your own needs. Then, reflect on what you require emotionally, mentally, and physically to heal and move forward. This may include a listening ear, reassurance, companionship, or practical assistance. Being self-aware and honest about what you need during this vulnerable time is essential.

Once you have identified your needs, communicate them honestly and directly to your support system. People cannot provide the support you need if they are unaware of what you're going through or the specific help you require. Be open and transparent about your feelings, concerns, and desires for support. Avoid bottling up your emotions or expecting others to guess what you need. Instead, clearly express your needs for understanding, validation, advice, or a shoulder to lean on. Honest communication fosters deeper connections and enables your support network to meet your needs more effectively.

Furthermore, be willing to accept and receive the support offered to you. Sometimes, after leaving a toxic relationship, you may feel unworthy of help or struggle with vulnerability. However, it's important to recognize that you deserve support and that accepting it does not make you weak or dependent. Allow yourself to be open to the caring gestures and assistance your support system provides. Getting help is not a burden but a testament to the strength and resilience it takes to acknowledge and seek support.

In summary, being honest about your needs is essential in keeping supportive people around you after leaving a toxic relationship. Take the time to identify and understand your own needs, then communicate them honestly and directly to your support system. Avoid expecting others to guess what you need and be open to accepting the support offered to you. By being honest and receptive, you create an environment of trust and understanding that fosters solid relationships and allows your support system to effectively provide the assistance you need to heal and gain closure.

Make time for them.

Being available for your support system is crucial in keeping supportive people around you after getting out of a toxic relationship. Firstly, prioritize your relationships by allocating dedicated time and attention to nurture them. Schedule regular check-ins or meet-ups with your supportive friends, family, or support group members. This consistent connection allows you to maintain a strong bond and ensures that your relationships remain a priority. By actively making time for your support system, you demonstrate your commitment to keeping them close and valued in your healing journey.

Secondly, be present and engaged during your interactions with your support system. When you spend time with them, please give them your full attention and actively listen to what they say. Engage in meaningful conversations, share your experiences, and ask about their well-being. Show genuine interest in their lives and provide support to them when they need it. Being present and engaged fosters a sense of reciprocity and strengthens the foundation of trust and care within your support system.

Lastly, be flexible and understanding in accommodating the schedules and needs of your support system. Recognize that everyone has their responsibilities and commitments. Offer flexibility when finding mutually convenient times to connect or meet. Be understanding if they cannot always be available immediately or need to reschedule due to prior commitments. You show respect and appreciation for their time and obligations by demonstrating flexibility and understanding. This fosters a positive and supportive dynamic within your relationships, ensuring your support system remains strong and present.

In summary, being available for your support system is vital in keeping supportive people around you after leaving a toxic relationship. Prioritize your relationships by scheduling regular check-ins or meet-ups. Be present and engaged during your interactions, actively listening and showing genuine interest. Accommodate the schedules and needs of your support system, offering flexibility and understanding. By actively investing time and effort into your relationships, you nurture a robust support system that remains by your side throughout your healing journey, providing the care and supports you need to gain closure and move forward healthily and positively.

Practice self-care.

Practicing self-care is essential in keeping supportive people around you after getting out of a toxic relationship. Firstly, prioritize your well-being by engaging in activities that promote self-care and self-nurturing. This can include engaging in hobbies or activities that bring you joy, practicing mindfulness or meditation, exercising regularly, getting enough sleep, and maintaining a balanced diet. Taking care of your physical, mental, and emotional health sends a powerful message to your support system that you value yourself and your needs. It also allows you to show up as your best self in your relationships, strengthening the bond between you and your supportive network.

Secondly, set boundaries to protect your energy and emotional well-being. Establish clear limits with others and communicate your needs openly. Be mindful of what you can and cannot handle, and assertively communicate your boundaries to your support system. This may include expressing the demand for space, asking for privacy, or stating what support you need. Setting and maintaining boundaries creates a healthy and balanced relationship dynamic where self-care and well-being are respected and prioritized.

Lastly, practice self-compassion and self-forgiveness. Understand that healing from a toxic relationship takes time and is not linear. Be kind to yourself and acknowledge that you are doing your best. Treat yourself with love, patience, and understanding, especially during difficult or setbacks. By practicing self-compassion, you cultivate a sense of self-worth and inner strength that radiates into your relationships. It allows your support system to see your resilience and encourages them to continue supporting and uplifting you in your journey.

In summary, practicing self-care is vital in keeping supportive people around you after leaving a toxic relationship. Prioritize your well-being through activities that promote self-care and self-nurturing. Set boundaries to protect your energy and emotional well-being and communicate your needs openly. Finally, practice self-compassion and self-forgiveness, recognizing that healing is a process. By caring for yourself, setting boundaries, and practicing self-compassion, you create a solid foundation for your relationships and ensure that supportive individuals remain present, providing the care and support you need to heal and thrive.

Seek out therapy.

Seeking out therapy or professional assistance is valuable in keeping supportive people around you after getting out of a toxic relationship. Firstly, therapy provides a safe and confidential space to process your emotions, heal from the trauma of toxic relationships, and develop healthy coping mechanisms. Treatment allows you to work through emotional wounds and gain clarity and insight into your experiences. By seeking professional help, you demonstrate a proactive approach to your healing journey, which can be reassuring to your support system. It shows that you are committed to your growth and well-being and can provide them with peace of mind knowing that you have the guidance and support of a trained professional.

Secondly, therapy can equip you with the tools and strategies to effectively communicate your needs and navigate the complexities of your relationships. A therapist can help you develop healthy boundaries, enhance communication skills, and navigate challenging dynamics. By learning these skills, you can cultivate more beneficial relationships with your support system and foster open, honest communication. This can lead to a deeper understanding and connection with those around you, strengthening the support system you have in place.

Lastly, therapy or professional assistance can help you address any lingering self-doubt, low self-esteem, or trust issues that may have resulted from the toxic relationship. You can rebuild your self-confidence, learn to trust again and work on unresolved trauma through treatment. This process of personal growth and healing can positively impact your relationships and allow you to show up more authentically and confidently with your support system. It can also help you identify and address any codependent patterns that may have developed during the toxic relationship, allowing you to cultivate healthier and more balanced relationships moving forward.

In summary, seeking therapy or professional assistance is instrumental in keeping supportive people around you after leaving a toxic relationship. Therapy provides a safe space to heal, gain insight, and develop healthy coping mechanisms. It equips you with the tools to communicate effectively and navigate complex dynamics within your relationships. Therapy also helps address self-esteem, trust issues, and any lingering trauma, allowing you to show up more confidently and authentically in your support system. You create a solid foundation for maintaining and strengthening your supportive network by prioritizing your mental and emotional well-being through therapy.

Join a support group.

Joining a support group is beneficial in keeping supportive people around you after getting out of a toxic relationship. Firstly, support groups provide a space where individuals who have gone through similar experiences can come together to share their stories, emotions, and insights. By joining a support group, you connect with people who understand and empathize with your journey, creating a sense of validation and belonging. The shared experiences within the group can foster a supportive community offering guidance, encouragement, and a listening ear. This support network can become integral to your healing process, ensuring you have a group of understanding individuals to turn to during challenging times.

Secondly, support groups offer a platform for learning and growth. Within these groups, you can gain insights and perspectives from others who have successfully navigated their healing journeys. The group discussions and interactions can provide valuable knowledge, coping strategies, and practical advice. You may learn about new resources, therapeutic techniques, or self-care practices that can enhance your healing process. By actively participating and engaging in the support group, you receive support and contribute to the approval of others, creating a reciprocal and empowering dynamic.

Lastly, support groups can help you build new and healthy relationships with individuals who share similar goals and values. As you interact with group members, you can form new friendships and connections based on mutual understanding and support. These relationships can extend beyond the support group meetings, providing you with ongoing companionship and encouragement. By forging new relationships within the support group, you expand your support network and create a sense of community that can continue to uplift you long after leaving the toxic relationship.

In summary, joining a support group is a valuable way to keep supportive people around you after getting out of a toxic relationship. Support groups provide a space for sharing experiences, receiving validation, and building connections with individuals who understand your journey. They offer opportunities for learning, growth and exchanging practical advice. Support groups also foster new and healthy relationships that can extend beyond the group meetings, creating a sense of community and ongoing support. By actively participating in a support group, you ensure you have a network of supportive individuals who can uplift, guide, and walk alongside you as you heal and gain closure.

Set boundaries.

Setting boundaries is crucial in keeping supportive people around you after getting out of a toxic relationship. Firstly, take the time to identify and establish your boundaries. Next, reflect on your needs, values, and limits, such as personal space, emotional well-being, and communication. Then, clearly define what is acceptable, and be firm in your decisions. Setting boundaries allows you to protect your energy and well-being, telling others that you value yourself and expect to be treated respectfully. It also helps you establish a sense of autonomy and regain control over your life, which is essential after leaving a toxic relationship.

Secondly, communicate your boundaries to your support system clearly and assertively. Let them know what you are comfortable with and what you are not. Be open and honest about your needs and expectations. Effective communication is vital in ensuring that your boundaries are understood and respected. Remember that it's okay to advocate for yourself and assert your limits. Those who truly support you will respect your boundaries and adjust their behavior accordingly. Setting and communicating boundaries creates a healthier relationship dynamic where your well-being is prioritized and upheld.

Lastly, enforce your boundaries consistently and with confidence. Stand firm in your decisions and hold others accountable for respecting your boundaries. It's natural for people to test limits occasionally, mainly if they were not accustomed to respecting them in the past. However, by consistently enforcing your boundaries, you show others you are serious about maintaining them. Be prepared to assertively and respectfully reiterate your boundaries if they are violated. This process of boundary enforcement can help filter out individuals who may not be supportive or respectful of your needs while also strengthening the relationships with those who genuinely care for your well-being.

In summary, setting boundaries is essential in keeping supportive people around you after leaving a toxic relationship. First, take the time to identify and establish your boundaries, clearly defining what is acceptable and what is not. Next, communicate your boundaries to your support system clearly and assertively. Finally, enforce your boundaries consistently and confidently, holding others accountable for respecting them. By setting and maintaining boundaries, you create a healthier and more respectful dynamic within your relationships, ensuring that supportive individuals remain present and respectful of your needs as you heal and move forward.

Express gratitude.

Expressing gratitude is a powerful way to keep supportive people around you after getting out of a toxic relationship. Firstly, take the time to reflect on the individuals who have been there for you during your healing process. Recognize their support, kindness, and understanding. Expressing gratitude acknowledges their efforts and reinforces the positive aspects of your relationships. It reminds you and your support system of their value and impact on your well-being. By expressing gratitude, you create a positive and appreciative atmosphere within your relationships, fostering a sense of connection and deepening the bond with those who have supported you.

Secondly, be specific and heartfelt when expressing your gratitude. Take the time to identify and articulate the particular ways in which individuals have helped you. It could be a listening ear, practical assistance, or emotional support. Be genuine in your expression, letting them know how their actions have made a difference in your life. This level of specificity and authenticity enhances the impact of your gratitude and makes the individuals feel seen and valued. It also encourages them to continue supporting and being present for you as you navigate your healing journey.

Lastly, express gratitude regularly and consistently. Make it a habit to acknowledge and appreciate the efforts of your support system. This can be done through verbal expressions, handwritten notes, or acts of kindness. Consistently expressing gratitude helps nurture relationships with supportive individuals and maintains a positive and uplifting dynamic. It serves as a reminder that their support is meaningful and appreciated. By consistently expressing gratitude, you create an environment where people feel valued and motivated to continue being a source of support for you.

In summary, expressing gratitude is a powerful way to keep supportive people around you after leaving a toxic relationship. Take the time to reflect on and acknowledge the individuals who have supported you during your healing journey. Be specific and heartfelt in expressing your gratitude, highlighting how they have made a positive impact. Express gratitude regularly and consistently to maintain a positive and appreciative atmosphere within your relationships. By expressing gratitude, you reinforce the value of your support system and encourage them to remain present and supportive as you gain closure and move forward healthily and positively.

Be open to new relationships.

Being open to new relationships is critical to keeping supportive people around you after getting out of a toxic relationship. Firstly, embrace the opportunity to meet new people and form connections. Next, recognize that not all relationships are unhealthy; some can bring positivity, understanding, and support into your life. By being open to new relationships, you expand your support network and create opportunities for meaningful connections with individuals who share your values and can contribute to your well-being. This openness allows you to cultivate healthy and supportive relationships vital to healing and closure.

Secondly, approach new relationships with a sense of discernment and self-awareness. Take the lessons from your toxic relationship and apply them to your interactions with others. Be mindful of red flags or patterns reminiscent of past toxic dynamics. Trust your instincts and prioritize your well-being. By being discerning and self-aware, you can make informed choices about the people you allow into your life, ensuring that they align with your values and contribute positively to your healing journey.

Lastly, communicate openly and honestly with new individuals in your life. Share your experiences and concerns, being transparent about your healing process. This vulnerability fosters deeper connections and attracts supportive, understanding, compassionate, and compassionate individuals. Communicating openly creates a foundation of trust and authenticity within your relationships. This allows you to build a network of supportive people willing to listen, offer guidance, and be there for you as you heal and gain closure.

In summary, being open to new relationships is essential in keeping supportive people around you after leaving a toxic relationship. Embrace the opportunity to meet new people and form connections, recognizing that healthy and positive relationships exist. Approach new relationships with discernment and self-awareness, learning from past experiences and prioritizing your well-being. Communicate openly and honestly with unique individuals, fostering trust and authenticity. By being open to new relationships, you expand your support network, cultivate healthy connections, and create a supportive community that uplifts and encourages your healing journey. Once out of an unhealthy relationship, you must maintain healthy relationships. It is essential to prioritize these individuals and their contributions to your well-being. Make time for them, express gratitude, and practice self-care. It's also important to set boundaries and communicate your discomfort. Finally, be open to new relationships and growth opportunities, as building and maintaining supportive relationships is ongoing. By taking these steps, you can create a robust support system to help you navigate healing challenges after a toxic relationship.

Step 8: How to Redefine Personal Happiness

After getting out of a toxic relationship, redefining personal happiness can seem daunting, but it is an essential step toward healing and moving forward. To do this, a person can start by reflecting on their needs and values and identifying the things that bring them joy and fulfillment. It is also important to practice self-care, surround oneself with positive and supportive people, set achievable goals, and focus on gratitude and forgiveness. Additionally, trying new hobbies or reconnecting with old friends or family members can help to broaden one's experiences and perspective. Through these steps and ongoing self-reflection, a person can create a new definition of happiness that aligns with their authentic self and sets the foundation for healthy, fulfilling relationships in the future.

Identify and prioritize your values:

Identifying and prioritizing your values is important in redefining personal happiness after getting out of a toxic relationship. Firstly, take the time to reflect on what truly matters to you in life. Next, consider the qualities, principles, and beliefs that guide your actions and decisions. These can range from integrity and compassion to personal growth and independence. By identifying your values, you understand what fulfills you and aligns with your authentic self. This clarity is a compass for navigating relationships, making choices, and pursuing activities that resonate with your core values.

Secondly, prioritize your values by intentionally incorporating them into your daily life. Once you have identified your values, consciously make decisions and set goals that align with them. For example, if personal growth is valuable, you may prioritize learning new skills or engaging in self-development activities. Living by your values creates a sense of purpose and fulfillment independent of external factors or toxic relationships. This shift in focus allows you to redefine personal happiness based on your values and aspirations rather than relying on the validation or approval of others.

Lastly, be open to revisiting and redefining your values as you grow and evolve. It is natural for values to shift or change over time, especially after experiencing a toxic relationship. Allow yourself the freedom to explore new perspectives, interests, and priorities. This flexibility enables personal growth and allows you to adapt your definition of happiness as you gain new insights and experiences. By continuously evaluating and redefining your values, you ensure that your pursuit of personal happiness remains aligned with your authentic self and reflects your evolving aspirations and desires.

In summary, identifying and prioritizing your values is vital in redefining personal happiness after leaving a toxic relationship. First, reflect on what truly matters to you and identify the qualities, principles, and beliefs that guide your life. Next, prioritize your values by incorporating them into your daily decisions and goals. This allows you to align with your core values, bringing a sense of purpose and fulfillment to your life. Finally, remain open to revisiting and redefining your values as you grow and evolve. By prioritizing your values, you create a foundation for personal happiness independent of toxic relationships and grounded in your authentic self.

Practice self-care.

Practicing self-care is crucial in redefining personal happiness after getting out of a toxic relationship. Firstly, prioritize your physical well-being by engaging in activities that promote self-nurturing and rejuvenation. This can include regular exercise, getting enough sleep, and maintaining a balanced diet. Taking care of your physical health boosts your energy and mood and empowers you to reclaim control over your body, which may have been compromised in a toxic relationship. By prioritizing self-care, you lay the foundation for overall well-being and set yourself up for a positive and fulfilling journey toward personal happiness.

Secondly, prioritize your emotional and mental well-being through self-reflection, mindfulness, and seeking support. Take time to reflect on your emotions, thoughts, and experiences, allowing yourself to process and heal from the toxicity you have endured. Engage in journaling, meditation, or therapy to cultivate self-awareness and emotional resilience. Addressing

12 Steps to Recovering from A Toxic Relationship

any lingering trauma, building coping mechanisms, and nurturing a positive mindset are important. Seeking support from trusted friends, family, or professionals can also be instrumental in your healing journey. By practicing self-care in this realm, you actively nurture your emotional well-being, foster resilience, and cultivate a positive mindset, all essential in redefining personal happiness.

Lastly, incorporate activities that bring joy, fulfillment, and a sense of purpose. Engage in hobbies, explore new interests, and set meaningful goals that align with your values and aspirations. Allow yourself to pursue activities that ignite your passion and creative fulfillment. This may involve creative endeavors, volunteering, or seeking personal growth opportunities. By actively engaging in activities that resonate with your authentic self, you create a fulfilling and purposeful life independent of toxic relationships. This self-care practice enables you to redefine personal happiness by focusing on what brings you joy and fulfillment, cultivating a sense of purpose and satisfaction.

Practicing self-care is vital in redefining personal happiness after leaving a toxic relationship. First, prioritize your physical well-being by engaging in activities that promote self-nurturing. Second, take care of your emotional and mental well-being through self-reflection, mindfulness, and seeking support. Third, incorporate activities that bring you joy, fulfillment, and a sense of purpose into your life. Practicing self-care in these areas fosters overall well-being, cultivates resilience, and creates a fulfilling and purpose-driven life independent of toxic relationships. Through self-care, you can redefine personal happiness on your terms and pave the way for a brighter and more fulfilling future.

Explore new hobbies or interests.

Exploring new hobbies or interests is a beautiful way to redefine personal happiness after getting out of a toxic relationship. Firstly, take the opportunity to discover activities that genuinely ignite your passion and curiosity. Then, explore by trying out different hobbies or interests you may have been curious about. This could include painting, dancing, playing an instrument, gardening, or exploring outdoor activities. By exploring new hobbies or interests, you open yourself up to new experiences, challenges, and opportunities for personal growth. This process allows you to rediscover yourself, your passions, and what brings you joy.

Secondly, fully immerse yourself in these new hobbies or interests. Dedicate time and energy to developing your skills and knowledge in the most intriguing areas. This commitment allows you to experience a sense of progress, accomplishment, and fulfillment. Engaging in activities that bring you joy creates a space for personal happiness independent of past toxic relationships. Exploring new hobbies or interests nurtures your individuality, boosts your self-esteem, and cultivates a sense of purpose and fulfillment.

Consider joining communities or groups related to your newfound hobbies or interests. Surrounding yourself with like-minded individuals who share your passions can be incredibly enriching and supportive. It provides an opportunity to connect, make new friends, and share experiences. Engaging with a community that shares your interests allows you to build a support network of individuals who uplift and inspire you. This sense of belonging can be instrumental in redefining personal happiness, as it fosters connections with people who appreciate and encourage your journey of self-discovery and growth.

In summary, exploring new hobbies or interests is a powerful way to redefine personal happiness after leaving a toxic relationship. Engage in self-exploration to discover activities that genuinely ignite your passion and curiosity. Fully immerse yourself in these new hobbies or interests, dedicating time and energy to develop your skills and knowledge. Consider joining communities or groups related to your newfound interests, allowing you to connect with like-minded individuals who share your passions. Through exploration, immersion, and community engagement, you create a space for personal happiness independent of toxic relationships, fostering personal growth, fulfillment, and a sense of purpose.

Set achievable goals for yourself.

Setting achievable goals for yourself is an effective way to redefine personal happiness after getting out of a toxic relationship. Firstly, take the time to reflect on what you want to achieve in different areas of your life, such as career, relationships, personal growth, and well-being. Then, start by setting small, manageable goals that align with your values and aspirations. These goals can be as simple as establishing a daily self-care routine, enrolling in a course or workshop to enhance your skills, or reconnecting with old friends. Setting achievable goals creates a sense of purpose and direction in your life, allowing you to work towards a happier and more fulfilling future actively.

Secondly, break down your larger goals into smaller, actionable steps. This helps to make them more attainable and less overwhelming. For example, suppose your goal is to start a new career. In that case, you can break it down into smaller steps, such as researching potential industries, updating your resume, networking, and applying for relevant job opportunities. By breaking goals into manageable steps, you create a clear roadmap for success and increase your chances of accomplishing them. Setting and achieving smaller goals contributes to progress and fulfillment, boosting your self-confidence and motivation to continue redefining personal happiness.

Lastly, celebrate your accomplishments along the way. Acknowledge and reward yourself for reaching milestones, no matter how small they may seem.

Celebrating your achievements reinforces a positive mindset and encourages you to keep progressing. It serves as a reminder of your growth and resilience, reminding you that you can overcome challenges and achieve the goals you set for yourself. By celebrating your progress, you create a positive feedback loop that fuels your motivation and reinforces your ability to redefine personal happiness on your terms.

Setting achievable goals for yourself is a powerful way to redefine personal happiness after leaving a toxic relationship. First, reflect on what you want to achieve and set small, manageable goals that align with your values and aspirations. Then, break down larger goals into actionable steps to make them more attainable and less overwhelming. Finally, celebrate your accomplishments to reinforce a positive mindset and keep your motivation high. By setting and achieving goals, you regain a sense of purpose, direction, and fulfillment, ultimately redefining personal happiness on your terms.

Surround yourself with positive and supportive people.

Surrounding yourself with positive and supportive people is crucial in redefining personal happiness after getting out of a toxic relationship. First, evaluate your social circle and identify those who uplift and support you. Then, focus on cultivating more profound connections with these individuals who positively impact your well-being. Next, seek friends, family members, or mentors who demonstrate empathy, understanding, and encouragement. You create a nurturing environment that fosters personal growth and happiness by surrounding yourself with positive and supportive people.

Secondly, set boundaries with toxic or negative individuals. It is essential to distance yourself from people who bring toxicity or drain your energy. This may involve creating healthy boundaries, limiting interactions, or cutting ties with individuals who consistently undermine your well-being. Creating distance from toxic influences allows you to create space for positive relationships to thrive and will enable you to prioritize your happiness and growth. Surrounding yourself with positive and supportive people means consciously investing your time and energy in relationships that positively contribute to your life.

Lastly, seek new connections and communities that align with your values and interests. Engage in activities, groups, or organizations that resonate with your passions and aspirations. This can be through joining clubs, attending events, or participating in hobbies that attract like-minded individuals. By immersing yourself in communities that share your values, you open up to new friendships and support networks. Surrounding yourself with people who share similar interests and goals creates a sense of belonging and provides a platform for personal growth and happiness. These positive connections can inspire and motivate you as you redefine your personal pleasure after a toxic relationship.

12 Steps to Recovering from A Toxic Relationship

In summary, surrounding yourself with positive and supportive people is vital in redefining personal happiness after leaving a toxic relationship. Evaluate your current social circle and focus on nurturing deeper connections with those who uplift and support you. Set boundaries with toxic individuals to create space for positive relationships to flourish. Actively seek new connections and communities aligning with your values and interests. By surrounding yourself with positive and supportive people, you create a nurturing environment that fosters personal growth, happiness, and a sense of belonging.

Practice gratitude.

Practicing gratitude is a powerful tool for redefining personal happiness after getting out of a toxic relationship. Firstly, cultivate a daily gratitude practice by taking a few moments each day to reflect on what you are grateful for. This can be done through journaling, making a gratitude list, or simply expressing gratitude in your thoughts. Next, please focus on the positive aspects of your life, no matter how small they may seem. By consciously acknowledging and appreciating the blessings, joys, and supportive people in your life, you shift your perspective towards gratitude, promoting personal happiness and contentment.

Secondly, practice gratitude in challenging situations. When faced with difficulties or setbacks, consciously look for silver linings or lessons to be learned. Rather than dwelling on the negative aspects of your past toxic relationship, focus on the tasks and growth opportunities that emerged from the experience. Expressing gratitude for the lessons learned, and the strength you gained empowers you to move forward and redefine your happiness. By reframing challenging situations through gratitude, you cultivate resilience, optimism, and a greater appreciation for the journey of self-discovery.

Lastly, express gratitude towards yourself. Recognize and celebrate your strengths, resilience, and progress. Acknowledge your steps to heal, grow, and move forward from the toxic relationship. Practice self-compassion and kindness towards yourself, appreciating your worth and value. You enhance your self-esteem and sense of self-worth by expressing gratitude for who you are and your journey. This, in turn, contributes to a deep understanding of personal happiness and fulfillment.

In summary, gratitude is a transformative practice in redefining personal happiness after leaving a toxic relationship. Cultivate a daily gratitude practice to focus on the positive aspects of your life. Practice gratitude in challenging situations, finding lessons and silver linings. Express gratitude towards yourself, acknowledging your strengths and celebrating your progress. Through gratitude, you shift your perspective, nurture a positive mindset, and cultivate a deep sense of personal happiness and contentment.

12 Steps to Recovering from A Toxic Relationship

Practice forgiveness:

Practicing forgiveness is a powerful and transformative way to redefine personal happiness after getting out of a toxic relationship. Firstly, it's important to understand that forgiveness is not about condoning or forgetting the hurt caused by the toxic relationship. Instead, it is a personal choice to release the negative emotions and resentment that may hold you back. Start by acknowledging your pain and allowing yourself to feel and process the emotions that arise. Then, make a conscious decision to let go of the past and forgive yourself and the other person involved. This forgiveness frees you from the emotional burden and creates space for healing and personal happiness.

Secondly, practice self-forgiveness. Often, individuals who have been in toxic relationships blame themselves for the circumstances or the choices they made. It is essential to recognize that you deserve forgiveness and compassion. Reflect on the lessons learned from the experience and acknowledge that you did the best you could with the knowledge and resources you had at the time. By practicing self-forgiveness, you release self-judgment and embrace self-love and acceptance. This allows you to redefine personal happiness by cultivating a positive and nurturing relationship with yourself.

Lastly, extend forgiveness to others involved in the toxic relationship. This includes forgiving the person who caused you harm and anyone else who may have played a role. Forgiveness does not mean that you have to reconcile or maintain a relationship with them, but rather it is a way to release the resentment and bitterness that may be holding you back. It is a process of letting go of negative emotions and finding peace within yourself. By practicing forgiveness, you break the cycle of anger and resentment, freeing yourself from the past and creating space for personal growth, happiness, and positive relationships in the future.

In summary, forgiveness is a transformative practice in redefining personal happiness after leaving a toxic relationship. Choose to release the negative emotions and resentment towards yourself and the others involved. Practice self-forgiveness by acknowledging your worth and embracing self-love and acceptance. Extend forgiveness to those who caused harm, freeing yourself from anger and resentment. Through forgiveness, you create space for healing, personal growth, and a renewed sense of happiness and well-being.

12 Steps to Recovering from A Toxic Relationship

Reconnect with old friends or family members.

Reconnecting with old friends or family members can be a valuable step in redefining personal happiness after getting out of a toxic relationship. Firstly, take the initiative to reach out to those who have been supportive and nurturing. Reconnecting with old friends or family members who have known you for a long time can provide a sense of familiarity, comfort, and understanding. In addition, these individuals may remind you of who you were before the toxic relationship and can help reignite your sense of self and personal happiness.

Secondly, be open and vulnerable when reconnecting with old friends or family members. Please share your experiences and emotions honestly, allowing them to understand your journey and provide the support you need. Rekindling connections with people who genuinely care about your well-being creates a safe space for healing and growth. By sharing your story and receiving empathy and validation, you nurture a sense of belonging and strengthen your support system, contributing to your happiness and well-being.

Lastly, actively engage in activities and create shared experiences with your old friends or family. Plan outings, gatherings, or virtual meetups to spend quality time together. Participate in activities you enjoy and promote a positive and uplifting environment. These shared experiences foster connection, laughter, and joy, allowing you to create new memories that replace the negative experiences from the toxic relationship.

Reconnecting with old friends or family members will enable you to rebuild and deepen relationships that contribute to your happiness and fulfillment.

In summary, reconnecting with old friends or family members can significantly redefine personal happiness after leaving a toxic relationship. Take the initiative to reach out to supportive individuals from your past. Be open and vulnerable when sharing your experiences and emotions. Engage in activities and create shared experiences that foster connection, laughter, and joy. You can rebuild and strengthen your support system through these reconnections, creating a nurturing environment that promotes personal growth, happiness, and a sense of belonging.

Seek professional counseling or therapy.

Seeking professional counseling or therapy is crucial in redefining personal happiness after getting out of a toxic relationship. Firstly, a qualified therapist or counselor can provide a safe and non-judgmental space to explore your emotions, heal from past wounds, and better understand yourself and your experiences. They can offer professional guidance and support, helping you navigate the complex emotions and challenges that arise during the healing process. Through therapy, you can gain valuable insights, develop coping strategies, and build resilience, which is essential in redefining personal happiness on your terms.

12 Steps to Recovering from A Toxic Relationship

Secondly, therapy can help you address any negative patterns or beliefs that may have developed due to the toxic relationship. A skilled therapist can assist you in identifying and challenging any self-limiting beliefs, negative self-talk, or unhealthy behaviors that may hinder your personal growth and happiness. They can help you develop healthier coping mechanisms, build self-esteem, and cultivate self-compassion. Working with a therapist can provide you with the tools and support necessary to break free from the cycle of toxicity and create a more fulfilling and balanced life.

Lastly, therapy offers a space for processing and healing from the emotional trauma that may have been inflicted during the toxic relationship. The therapeutic process allows you to validate your experiences, work through any unresolved feelings of anger, sadness, or betrayal, and ultimately find a sense of closure. By addressing and processing the emotional wounds, you can begin to let go of the pain and move forward with a renewed sense of personal happiness and well-being. Therapy provides a dedicated space and professional guidance to help you heal, grow, and redefine your happiness after a toxic relationship.

In summary, seeking professional counseling or therapy is valuable in redefining personal happiness after leaving a toxic relationship. A therapist can provide a safe and non-judgmental space for you to explore your emotions, gain insights, and develop coping strategies. Therapy can help address negative patterns, beliefs, and behaviors, fostering personal growth and resilience. It also offers an opportunity to process and heal from the emotional trauma associated with the toxic relationship. By working with a therapist, you can find support, guidance, and healing, ultimately paving the way for a happier and healthier future.

Take time to reflect.

Reflecting is essential in redefining personal happiness after getting out of a toxic relationship. Firstly, create a dedicated space for self-reflection where you can introspect and examine your emotions, thoughts, and experiences. This can be done through journaling, meditation, or simply finding a quiet place where you feel comfortable and at ease. Next, reflect on the lessons you have learned from the toxic relationship, the patterns that may have emerged, and the impact it had on your well-being. By gaining clarity through reflection, you can better understand yourself and what truly brings you happiness.

Secondly, use reflection as an opportunity to redefine your values and priorities. Take the time to identify what truly matters to you and align your actions and choices accordingly. Reflect on what makes you feel fulfilled, joyful, and at peace. Consider the activities, relationships, and experiences contributing to your happiness. By consciously reevaluating and redefining your values, you can make choices that align with your authentic self and create a life that reflects your true desires and aspirations.

12 Steps to Recovering from A Toxic Relationship

Lastly, reflect on your strengths and resilience. Acknowledge the progress you have made and the growth you have experienced throughout your journey. Recognize the courage it took to leave the toxic relationship and the steps you have taken to prioritize your well-being. Reflect on your worth and the qualities that make you unique and valuable. Focusing on your strengths and resilience can rebuild your self-confidence and create a strong foundation for personal happiness. Taking time to reflect allows you to gain self-awareness, redefine your values, and appreciate your growth and potential.

In summary, reflecting is a powerful practice for redefining personal happiness after leaving a toxic relationship. Create a dedicated space for self-reflection, allowing for introspection and examination of your emotions, thoughts, and experiences. Use reflection as an opportunity to redefine your values and priorities, aligning your actions and choices with what truly brings you happiness. Reflect on your strengths and resilience, acknowledging your progress and appreciating your worth. Through reflection, you can gain self-awareness, redefine your values, and cultivate a more profound sense of personal happiness and fulfillment. After getting out of a toxic relationship, redefining what happiness means and looks like can be challenging. It's important to remember that personal happiness is unique to each individual, and the journey toward it may take time and effort. Some possible steps to redefine personal happiness after leaving a toxic relationship include identifying and prioritizing personal values, practicing self-care, exploring new hobbies or interests, setting achievable goals, surrounding oneself with positive and supportive people, practicing gratitude and forgiveness, reconnecting with old friends or family members, seeking professional counseling or therapy, and taking time to reflect on one's personal growth and progress.

By taking these steps, individuals can gradually rebuild their sense of self, regain confidence and self-worth, and cultivate a fulfilling and joyful life. It's important to remember that this journey is a process, and there may be setbacks and challenges. However, redefining personal happiness and creating a fulfilling and joyful life is possible with patience, self-compassion, and a commitment to personal growth.

Step 9: Stay Grounded In Their Current Position

Getting out of a toxic relationship can be a challenging experience, and it's crucial to prioritize your mental and emotional well-being as you navigate this transition. One way to do this is by staying grounded in your current position, which means staying connected to your sense of self and finding stability and balance in your daily life. This can help you feel more secure, confident, and in control, which is essential for moving forward in a positive direction and avoiding falling back into old patterns or relationships that may not serve you. By staying grounded, you can set the stage for a brighter, healthier future filled with opportunities for growth, self-discovery, and happiness.

Practice self-care:

Practicing self-care is crucial to staying grounded in your current position after getting out of a toxic relationship. Firstly, prioritize your physical well-being by engaging in activities that promote self-nurturing. Establish a regular exercise routine that suits your preferences and abilities, as physical activity has been proven to reduce stress and improve overall well-being. Additionally, maintain a balanced and nutritious diet, as fueling your body with healthy foods can positively impact your energy levels and mood. Engaging in yoga, meditation, or deep breathing exercises can also help reduce stress and promote a sense of inner calm and stability.

Secondly, focus on nurturing your emotional well-being by engaging in activities that bring you joy and relaxation. Engage in hobbies or activities you love, whether reading, painting, gardening, or listening to music. Prioritize activities that help you unwind and recharge, such as relaxing baths, walking in nature, or spending quality time with loved ones. Additionally, set boundaries and prioritize self-care by saying no to activities or commitments that drain your energy or do not align with your well-being. By caring for your emotional needs and engaging in activities that bring you happiness and fulfillment, you can stay grounded and centered in your current position.

Lastly, don't forget to nurture your mental well-being by practicing self-compassion and mindfulness. Be kind and patient with yourself as you navigate the healing process. Challenge negative self-talk and replace it with positive affirmations and self-empowering beliefs. Cultivate mindfulness by being present and observing your thoughts and emotions without judgment. Engaging in mindfulness practices, such as meditation or mindful breathing, can help you stay grounded and maintain a sense of inner peace. Prioritizing your mental well-being through self-compassion and mindfulness practices allows you to navigate any challenges that may arise and stay grounded in your current position.

In summary, practicing self-care is essential for staying grounded in your current position after leaving a toxic relationship. First, prioritize your physical well-being through regular exercise, a balanced diet, and engaging in activities that promote relaxation. Next, nurture your emotional well-being by participating in activities that bring joy and setting boundaries to prioritize self-care. Lastly, nurture your mental well-being through self-compassion and mindfulness practices. By practicing self-care, you can maintain stability and inner peace and remain grounded in your current position as you continue healing and personal growth.

Build a support network.

Building a support network is essential for staying grounded in your current position after getting out of a toxic relationship. Firstly, reach out to trusted friends and family members who can provide emotional support and understanding. Please share your experiences and feelings with them, allowing them to offer guidance, validation, and a listening ear. These supportive individuals can help you process your emotions, provide perspective, and remind you of your strength and resilience. In addition, building a support network of trusted loved ones creates a sense of belonging and community, which can help you stay grounded and connected during the healing process.

Secondly, consider seeking professional support through therapy or counseling. A trained therapist or counselor can provide a safe and confidential space to explore your emotions, gain insights, and develop coping strategies. They can offer guidance and support tailored to your specific needs and circumstances. Working with a professional can provide you with an objective perspective, help you navigate the challenges that arise, and offer tools for self-care and personal growth. Building a support network that includes professional assistance ensures you have access to specialized expertise and resources to further your journey of staying grounded.

Lastly, consider joining support groups or seeking out online communities of individuals who have experienced similar toxic relationships. These groups provide a space for shared experiences, empathy, and understanding. Engaging with others who have gone through similar challenges can provide validation, inspiration, and a sense of belonging. Support groups offer opportunities to learn from others, gain new perspectives, and receive guidance on staying grounded and moving forward. Building a support network with peers who can relate to your experiences can provide valuable camaraderie and support.

Building a support network is crucial for staying grounded in your current position after leaving a toxic relationship. Contact trusted friends and family, share your experiences, and seek their emotional support. Seek professional help through therapy or counseling to gain specialized guidance and support. Additionally, join support groups or online communities to connect with others who have experienced similar situations. Building a support network ensures you have a strong foundation of support, guidance, and understanding as

12 Steps to Recovering from A Toxic Relationship

you navigate the healing process and stay grounded in your current position.

Set boundaries.

Setting boundaries is crucial to staying grounded in your current position after getting out of a toxic relationship. Firstly, clearly define your limits and communicate them assertively to others. Next, identify what is acceptable and unacceptable to you regarding behavior, communication, and interactions. Finally, communicate your boundaries calmly and confidently, expressing your needs and expectations. By setting and communicating your boundaries, you establish a clear framework for how you want to be treated, which helps you maintain a sense of control and self-respect.

Secondly, be consistent in enforcing your boundaries. It's important to uphold your boundaries consistently, even when faced with resistance or pushback. This may require saying "no" to people or situations that violate your boundaries. It's natural for some individuals to test or challenge your boundaries, especially if they were not respected in the past. However, staying firm and consistent conveys that your boundaries are non-negotiable. By enforcing your boundaries, you protect your emotional well-being and maintain a sense of empowerment and self-worth.

Lastly, practice self-care as a boundary-setting tool. Prioritize self-care activities that recharge and nourish your mind, body, and soul. Make time for activities that bring you joy, relaxation, and peace. Setting boundaries around your self-care routines sends a message that your well-being is a priority and that you are committed to staying grounded. This may involve saying "no" to specific obligations or carving out dedicated time for yourself. By prioritizing self-care and setting boundaries around it, you create a foundation of self-nurturing and self-respect, contributing to your groundedness and well-being.

Setting boundaries is essential for staying grounded in your current position after leaving a toxic relationship. Clearly define and communicate your boundaries, expressing your needs and expectations to others. Be consistent in enforcing your boundaries, even in the face of resistance. Practice self-care as a boundary-setting tool, prioritizing activities that nourish and rejuvenate you. Setting and upholding your boundaries protects your emotional well-being, maintains a sense of control, and stays grounded in your current position.

Cultivate a positive mindset.

Cultivating a positive mindset is crucial for staying grounded in your current position after getting out of a toxic relationship. Firstly, practice self-awareness and monitor your thoughts. Notice any negative or self-limiting beliefs lingering from the toxic relationship and challenge them. Replace negative thoughts with positive affirmations and empowering beliefs. Focus on your strengths, resilience, and the progress you have made. By actively shifting your mindset towards positivity, you can reframe your perspective and cultivate a more optimistic outlook on life.

12 Steps to Recovering from A Toxic Relationship

Secondly, practice gratitude as a daily habit. Take time each day to reflect on what you are grateful for, no matter how small. This could be anything from a beautiful sunset to the support of loved ones or personal achievements. By actively cultivating gratitude, you shift your focus toward the positive aspects of your life and develop a sense of appreciation. This helps counteract negative emotions and keeps you grounded in the present moment.

Lastly, surround yourself with positive influences and inspirational resources. Seek books, podcasts, or videos promoting personal growth, resilience, and positivity. Engage with supportive communities or groups that uplift and encourage you. Surrounding yourself with positive influences helps reinforce your positive mindset and provides a supportive network of like-minded individuals. By consciously curating your environment and seeking positive resources, you can maintain a grounded perspective and stay motivated on your personal happiness and growth journey.

In summary, cultivating a positive mindset is vital for staying grounded in your current position after leaving a toxic relationship. First, practice self-awareness to monitor and challenge negative thoughts, replacing them with positive affirmations and empowering beliefs. Next, cultivate gratitude as a daily habit, focusing on what you are grateful for and shifting your perspective towards the positive aspects of life. Finally, surround yourself with positive influences and inspirational resources that support your personal growth and well-being. By cultivating a positive mindset, you can stay grounded, resilient, and open to new possibilities for personal happiness and fulfillment.

Find healthy coping methods.

Finding healthy coping methods is crucial for staying grounded in your current position after getting out of a toxic relationship. Firstly, it's important to prioritize self-care. This involves taking care of your physical, emotional, and mental well-being. Engage in activities that bring you joy and relaxation, such as practicing mindfulness, regular exercise, getting enough sleep, and nourishing your body with nutritious food. Self-care helps to reduce stress, promotes self-compassion, and allows you to recharge and rejuvenate.

Secondly, consider engaging in therapeutic activities for emotional expression and healing. This can include journaling, art therapy, or practicing deep breathing exercises. Journaling provides an outlet for processing your emotions, reflecting on your experiences, and gaining clarity. Art therapy, such as painting or drawing, can help you express and release pent-up emotions in a creative and non-verbal way. Finally, deep breathing exercises and mindfulness practices help to calm the mind and body, reducing anxiety and promoting relaxation.

Lastly, seek support from trusted friends, family, or support groups. Surrounding yourself with a supportive network of individuals who understand and validate your experiences can be invaluable. Share your feelings, thoughts, and concerns with them, and allow them to provide guidance and support. Support groups, either in-person or online, offer a safe space to connect with others who have gone through similar experiences, providing an opportunity to share and learn from one another.

In summary, finding healthy coping methods is essential for staying grounded after leaving a toxic relationship. Prioritize self-care by engaging in activities that promote your overall well-being. Explore therapeutic activities that allow for emotional expressions and healing, such as journaling, art therapy, or mindfulness practices. Seek support from trusted friends, family, or support groups to create a supportive network of individuals who can offer understanding and guidance. Finding healthy coping methods, you can navigate the healing process, maintain your groundedness, and move forward positively and healthily.

Practice forgiveness.

Practicing forgiveness is a powerful way to stay grounded in your current position after getting out of a toxic relationship. Firstly, it's important to understand that forgiveness is not about condoning or excusing the toxic behavior. Instead, it's a process of releasing yourself from the emotional burden and resentment that can hold you back. Recognize that forgiveness is a personal journey and may take time and effort. Begin by acknowledging your pain and allowing yourself to process the arising emotions. Journaling or speaking with a trusted friend or therapist can help facilitate this process.

Secondly, shift your perspective by practicing empathy and compassion towards yourself and the person who caused the harm. Understand that toxic behavior often stems from the person's unresolved issues and pain. This doesn't justify their actions, but it can help you see them as flawed human beings rather than solely as villains. Developing empathy towards yourself is equally important. Release any self-blame or guilt you may be carrying and remind yourself that you deserve healing and happiness. By cultivating compassion, you create space for forgiveness to grow.

Lastly, focus on personal growth and learning from the experience. Reflect on the lessons you've gained from the toxic relationship and use them as a catalyst for self-improvement. Identify the patterns and red flags you've encountered and commit to establishing healthy boundaries in future relationships. Embrace the opportunity to rediscover your values, priorities, and strengths. By focusing on personal growth, you empower yourself to move forward and stay grounded in your current position with a renewed sense of purpose and resilience.

In summary, practicing forgiveness is a transformative process that helps you stay grounded after leaving a toxic relationship. Begin by acknowledging your pain and allowing yourself to process the emotions involved. Next, shift your perspective by practicing empathy and compassion towards yourself and the person who caused the harm. Finally, focus on personal growth and learning from the experience to establish healthy boundaries and rediscover your strengths and values. By practicing forgiveness, you free yourself from the emotional burden of the past and create a solid foundation for staying grounded in your current position.

Learn from the experience.

Learning from experience is crucial for staying grounded in your current position after getting out of a toxic relationship. Firstly, reflect on the relationship dynamics and identify the red flags and patterns contributing to the toxicity. Next, assess what behaviors or situations led to the unhealthy dynamics and consider how you can recognize and avoid them in the future. This self-reflection allows you to gain valuable insights into yourself and your needs, empowering you to make more informed decisions.

Secondly, prioritize personal growth and self-development. Use the lessons learned from the toxic relationship as an opportunity to gain experience and evolve. Invest time and energy into understanding your values, boundaries, and priorities. Focus on building your self-esteem and self-confidence, as these qualities will help you establish healthier relationships in the future. Seek resources such as self-help books, therapy, or support groups to enhance your growth journey further. Embrace the learning process to empower yourself and create a solid foundation for your current position.

Lastly, practice self-care and self-compassion throughout your healing journey. Nurture your physical, emotional, and mental well-being by engaging in activities that bring joy, reduce stress, and promote self-care. Surround yourself with positive influences and supportive individuals who uplift and encourage you. Celebrate your progress and acknowledge the strength it took to leave the toxic relationship. By prioritizing self-care and self-compassion, you create a solid foundation of self-worth and resilience that will help you stay grounded in your current position.

In summary, learning from the experience is critical to staying grounded after getting out of a toxic relationship. Reflect on the dynamics and patterns that contributed to the toxicity and use this knowledge to recognize and avoid similar situations in the future. Prioritize personal growth and self-development to understand your values, boundaries, and priorities. Practice self-care and self-compassion to nurture your well-being and surround yourself with positive influences. By learning from the experience, you can create a strong foundation for staying grounded in your current position and building healthier, fulfilling relationships.

Find ways to stay connected to your passions.

Finding ways to stay connected to your passions is vital for staying grounded in your current position after getting out of a toxic relationship. Firstly, take the time to reconnect with yourself and identify the activities or hobbies that bring you joy and fulfillment. Next, reflect on the passions and interests that may have been neglected or suppressed during the toxic relationship. These activities allow you to rediscover your identity and reclaim your sense of self. Whether painting, playing a musical instrument, writing, or engaging in sports, find ways to incorporate your passions into your daily life.

Secondly, prioritize self-care and make your passions a non-negotiable part of your routine. Schedule dedicated time for your hobbies and passions, even if it means starting with small increments. Treat these activities as a form of self-care and self-expression, allowing yourself to fully immerse yourself in the present moment and find solace in your passions. Engaging in activities that you love can be therapeutic and serve as an outlet for emotional release. It helps to reduce stress, boost your mood, and provide a sense of accomplishment and fulfillment.

Lastly, explore new interests and expand your horizons. Use this transition period as an opportunity to explore and discover new passions. Try different activities, take classes or workshops, and step out of your comfort zone. Embrace the journey of self-discovery and allow yourself to be open to new experiences. Constantly seeking and nurturing your passions creates a sense of purpose, joy, and fulfillment that contributes to staying grounded in your current position.

In summary, finding ways to stay connected to your passions is essential for staying grounded after getting out of a toxic relationship. Take the time to reconnect with yourself and identify the activities that bring you joy and fulfillment. Prioritize self-care and make your passions a non-negotiable part of your routine. Explore new interests and embrace the journey of self-discovery. By staying connected to your passions, you create a sense of purpose, joy, and fulfillment that contributes to your overall well-being and helps you stay grounded in your current position.

Create a vision for your future.

Creating a vision for your future is a powerful way to stay grounded in your current position after getting out of a toxic relationship. Firstly, reflect on your values, dreams, and aspirations. What are the things that truly matter to you? What kind of life do you envision for yourself moving forward? Clarifying your vision helps establish a sense of direction and purpose, providing a solid foundation for your current position. Next, visualize your desired future and set goals that align with your vision.

Secondly, break down your vision into actionable steps. Once you have a clear picture of where you want to be, identify the smaller goals and milestones to help you progress toward your vision. These can be personal, professional, or relational goals. Make your goals specific, measurable, attainable, relevant, and time-bound (SMART goals). By breaking down your vision into manageable steps, you create a roadmap for success and stay grounded in your current position by consistently working towards your desired future.

12 Steps to Recovering from A Toxic Relationship

Lastly, stay flexible and open to the possibilities that may arise on your journey. While having a vision is important, remaining adaptable and embracing unexpected opportunities and challenges is equally crucial. Life is full of twists and turns, and staying grounded means being willing to adjust your path as needed. Cultivate resilience and a growth mindset, viewing obstacles as learning experiences and opportunities for personal development. By maintaining flexibility and an open mind, you can navigate the ups and downs of life while staying grounded in your current position and moving steadily toward your envisioned future.

In summary, creating a vision for your future is critical to staying grounded after getting out of a toxic relationship. First, reflect on your values and aspirations, and clarify the life you envision for yourself. Then, break down your vision into actionable steps, setting **"SMART"** goals that align with your desired future. Finally, stay flexible and open-minded, adapting to unexpected opportunities and challenges. By creating a vision for your future and working towards it, you cultivate a sense of purpose and direction that helps you stay grounded in your current position.

Celebrate your progress:

Celebrating your progress is an essential practice to stay grounded in your current position after getting out of a toxic relationship. Firstly, take the time to acknowledge and appreciate the steps you've taken and the milestones you've achieved along your healing journey. Recognize the strength and resilience it took to leave the toxic relationship and honor your progress since then. Celebrating your progress boosts your self-esteem and confidence, reminding you of your capabilities and empowering you to continue moving forward. Secondly, find meaningful ways to celebrate your achievements. It can be as simple as treating yourself to something you enjoy, such as a spa day, a special meal, or a small gift. You can also celebrate by sharing your accomplishments with loved ones, friends, or a support network that has been there for you throughout your healing process. Their acknowledgment and support can further reinforce your progress and validate your growth. Finally, celebrating your progress creates a positive and joyful atmosphere that encourages you to keep going and stay grounded in your current position. Lastly, keep a record of your achievements and milestones. Create a journal or a gratitude jar to document your progress and moments of pride. This allows you to reflect on how far you've come and is a tangible reminder of your growth and strength. When you face challenges or moments of doubt, revisit these records to remind yourself of your resilience and progress. Tangibly celebrating your progress provides a sense of fulfillment and encourages you to keep striving for personal growth and happiness.

In summary, celebrating your progress is crucial for staying grounded after getting out of a toxic relationship. Take the time to acknowledge and appreciate the steps you have taken and the milestones you've achieved. Find meaningful ways to celebrate, whether treating yourself or sharing your accomplishments with loved ones. Keep a record of your achievements to reflect on your growth and strength. By celebrating your progress, you reinforce your self-esteem, motivation, and determination to stay grounded in your current position and continue the path of healing and personal growth.

A toxic relationship can be a life-changing experience that leaves you feeling emotionally drained, confused, and disconnected from your sense of self. This is why staying grounded in your current position is so important. By staying grounded, you can find a sense of stability and balance in your life, which can help you rebuild your confidence and sense of self-worth. In addition, you can prioritize your mental and emotional well-being and focus on healing and moving forward positively.

****S.M.A.R.T. Goals****

SMART goals are a framework for setting specific, measurable, attainable, relevant, and time-bound objectives. Each letter in the acronym represents a critical element of practical goal setting.

S - Specific: A SMART goal should be clear and well-defined. It should answer the questions of who, what, where, when, why, and how. By being specific, you clearly understand what you want to achieve and can focus your efforts accordingly.

M - Measurable: A SMART goal should be quantifiable to track your progress and determine when you have achieved it. It involves identifying the metrics or criteria that will indicate your success. Having measurable goals allows you to stay motivated and provides a sense of accomplishment as you see tangible progress.

A - Attainable: A SMART goal should be challenging yet realistic and attainable. It should stretch you outside your comfort zone but remain within the realm of possibility. Setting too ambitious or unrealistic goals can lead to frustration and disappointment. By ensuring your goals are attainable, you set yourself up for success and maintain a sense of motivation and progress.

R- Relevant: A SMART goal should be relevant and aligned with your overall objectives and values. It should have significance and be meaningful to you. By setting goals pertinent to your broader aspirations, you maintain focus and ensure that your efforts contribute to your overall growth and fulfillment.

T - Time-Bound: A SMART goal should have a clear timeframe or deadline. It specifies when you expect to achieve the goal, providing a sense of urgency and accountability. A deadline helps you prioritize your actions and allocate your time and resources effectively. Setting a time-bound goal creates a sense of structure and commitment to achieving your objectives.

In summary, SMART goals are specific, measurable, attainable, relevant, and time-bound. They provide a framework for effective goal setting by ensuring clarity, measurability, feasibility, alignment, and a sense of urgency. By incorporating these elements into your goal-setting process, you increase the likelihood of success and stay focused and motivated to achieve your desired outcomes.

Keith L. Belvin

Step 10: How a Person Can Care For Themselves, Physically, Mentally, Emotionally, and Spiritually.

A toxic breakup can leave a person feeling drained, disoriented, and disconnected from themselves. During this challenging time, it's important to prioritize self-care in all areas of life, including physical, mental, emotional, and spiritual health. By caring for oneself in these ways, one can rebuild their sense of self-worth, find balance and stability, and set the stage for healing and growth. Taking time to care for oneself after a toxic breakup can help one navigate the complex emotions that arise, such as grief, anger, and confusion. It can also help them move forward positively with greater strength, clarity, and resilience.

Practice self-compassion:

Practicing self-compassion is crucial for caring for oneself holistically after getting out of a toxic relationship. Firstly, be gentle and kind to yourself, understanding that healing takes time and that you may still carry emotional wounds from the toxic relationship. Next, acknowledge and accept your emotions without judgment, allowing yourself to feel and process them. Finally, offer yourself compassion and self-soothing techniques, such as practicing mindfulness, deep breathing exercises, or engaging in activities that bring joy and peace. By treating yourself with kindness and understanding, you create a safe space for emotional healing and allow yourself to care for your mental and emotional well-being fully.

Secondly, prioritize self-care on a physical level. Please consider your body's needs and nurture them with healthy habits. Regularly exercise, eat nourishing foods, and get sufficient rest and sleep. Listen to your body's signals and take breaks when needed. Self-compassion involves honoring your physical boundaries and taking care of yourself in a way that promotes vitality and overall well-being. Engaging in activities that nourish your body, such as practicing yoga, walking in nature, or indulging in a soothing bath, can also contribute to your emotional and spiritual well-being.

Lastly, cultivate self-compassion on a spiritual level. Connect with your inner self and explore practices that nurture your spiritual growth. This can involve engaging in meditation, prayer, or other forms of introspection that align with your beliefs and values. Allow yourself to explore your spirituality in a way that feels authentic and meaningful. By nurturing your spiritual connection, you create a sense of inner peace, guidance, and resilience that can support you on your journey of healing and self-care.

In summary, practicing self-compassion is essential for caring for oneself holistically after getting out of a toxic relationship. Be gentle and kind to yourself, allowing emotional healing and processing space. Prioritize self-care on physical, mental, emotional, and spiritual levels, listening to your body's needs and engaging in activities that promote well-being. Cultivate self-compassion by nurturing your inner self and connecting with your spirituality. By practicing self-compassion, you create a foundation of self-care and self-love that supports your overall well-being after the end of a toxic relationship.

Take care of your physical health.

Taking care of your physical health is crucial for caring for yourself holistically after getting out of a toxic relationship. Firstly, prioritize regular exercise to boost your physical well-being. Engaging in physical activity releases endorphins, improving your mood and reducing stress. Next, find an exercise routine that suits your preferences and schedule, whether running, practicing yoga, or joining a fitness class. Finally, aim for consistency rather than intensity, focusing on activities that bring you joy and help you reconnect with your body. Regular exercise supports your physical health and contributes to your mental and emotional well-being.

Secondly, pay attention to your nutrition and nourish your body with wholesome foods. Opt for a balanced diet that includes a variety of fruits, vegetables, lean proteins, whole grains, and healthy fats. Prioritize foods that provide essential nutrients and promote overall well-being. Remember to hydrate properly by drinking adequate water throughout the day. Fueling your body with nutritious foods provides the energy and nutrients necessary to support your physical and mental health. It can also increase energy levels, mood, and overall functioning.

Lastly, prioritize rest and sleep to recharge your body and mind. Adequate sleep is essential for physical and mental well-being, allowing your body to repair and rejuvenate. Therefore, establish a consistent sleep schedule, create a relaxing bedtime routine, and ensure your sleep environment is comfortable and conducive to restful sleep. Additionally, practice stress management techniques, such as deep breathing exercises or meditation, to help calm your mind and promote relaxation. Getting enough restful sleep and managing stress supports your overall well-being and enhance your ability to care for yourself on all levels.

In summary, taking care of your physical health is vital for caring for yourself holistically after leaving a toxic relationship. Prioritize regular exercise to boost your mood and reduce stress. Pay attention to your nutrition and fuel your body with wholesome foods. Make sleep a priority and practice stress management techniques. By caring for your physical health, you create a foundation for self-care that supports your overall well-being and allows you to care for yourself physically, mentally, emotionally, and spiritually.

Find healthy ways to manage stress.

Finding healthy ways to manage stress is essential for caring for yourself holistically after getting out of a toxic relationship. Firstly, identify the stressors in your life and develop effective coping strategies. This could involve engaging in activities that help you relax and unwind, such as practicing mindfulness or meditation, engaging in hobbies you enjoy, or spending time in nature. These activities can help reduce stress, promote emotional well-being, and provide inner peace. Experiment with different stress management techniques to find what works best for you and make them a regular part of your self-care routine.

Secondly, prioritize self-care practices that promote stress relief. This could include taking regular daily breaks to engage in activities that bring you joy and relaxation. Whether reading a book, taking a warm bath, listening to music, or practicing deep breathing exercises, find activities that help you recharge and replenish your energy. Also, establish healthy personal and professional boundaries to manage stress more effectively. Say no to activities or commitments that overwhelm you and prioritize self-care without feeling guilty. Taking care of your needs and managing stress allows you to maintain your physical, mental, and emotional well-being.

Lastly, seek support from trusted friends, family, or professionals. Sharing your feelings and experiences with others who are supportive, and understanding can be incredibly therapeutic. Consider joining a support group or seeking therapy to process your emotions and gain valuable insights into managing stress. Professional guidance can provide practical strategies and tools to navigate challenges after leaving a toxic relationship. Surrounding yourself with a strong support network allows you to lean on others during difficult times and receive the encouragement and validation needed to care for yourself holistically.

In summary, finding healthy ways to manage stress is crucial for caring for yourself physically, mentally, emotionally, and spiritually after leaving a toxic relationship. First, identify stressors and develop effective coping strategies. Second, prioritize self-care practices that promote stress relief and establish healthy boundaries. Finally, seek support from trusted individuals or professionals who provide guidance and understanding. By managing stress healthily, you empower yourself to care for your overall well-being and navigate the healing journey with resilience and self-compassion.

Seek professional support.

Seeking professional support is an important step in caring for yourself holistically after getting out of a toxic relationship. Firstly, consider finding a therapist or counselor specializing in relationship trauma and healing. They can provide a safe and non-judgmental space to process your emotions, gain insights into your experiences, and develop coping strategies. In addition, a professional can offer guidance and support as you navigate the challenges of healing from a toxic relationship. They can also help you identify patterns, beliefs, and behaviors hindering your self-care and guide you toward healthier coping mechanisms.

Secondly, if you are experiencing symptoms of anxiety, depression, or trauma, consider consulting with a mental health professional. They can assess your mental health needs and provide appropriate interventions or treatments. This may include therapy techniques such as cognitive-behavioral therapy (CBT), eye movement desensitization and reprocessing, Eye movement desensitization and reprocessing (EMDR), or other evidence-based approaches that target trauma and its effects. Professional support can help you manage psychological distress, promote emotional healing, and provide valuable self-care and personal growth tools.

Lastly, consider seeking guidance from a spiritual or religious counselor if you have spiritual or religious beliefs that are important to you. They can offer support, guidance, and a listening ear as you navigate the spiritual aspects of your healing journey. This can involve exploring your values and beliefs and finding meaning in your experiences. In addition, spiritual or religious counselors can provide insights, rituals, and practices that align with your beliefs and support your spiritual well-being.

In summary, seeking professional support is crucial for caring for yourself physically, mentally, emotionally, and spiritually after leaving a toxic relationship. First, find a therapist or counselor specializing in relationship trauma to provide guidance and support in healing. Next, consider consulting with a mental health professional to address psychological distress. Finally, seek guidance from a spiritual or religious counselor to support your spiritual well-being. Professional support can give you the tools, insights, and validation to navigate your healing journey and care for yourself holistically.

Connect with supportive people.

Connecting with supportive people is vital for caring for yourself holistically after getting out of a toxic relationship. Firstly, identify individuals in your life who are supportive, understanding, and empathetic. This could be close friends, family members, or even support groups of individuals who have experienced similar situations. Surrounding yourself with people who uplift and validate you can provide a sense of belonging, reduce isolation, and create a supportive network that fosters your overall well-being.

Secondly, communicate your needs and boundaries to your support network. Let them know how they can best support you during this healing process. Whether having someone to talk to, asking for practical help, or simply seeking companionship, expressing your needs allows others to understand and provide the support you require. Additionally, set clear boundaries with toxic or unsupportive individuals to protect your emotional and mental well-being. Creating a safe space with supportive people who respect your boundaries is crucial for ongoing self-care.

Lastly, actively engage in activities and share experiences with your support network. Participate in social gatherings, hobbies, or group activities that bring joy and foster a sense of connection. This could include joining clubs or organizations centered around your interests or attending support group meetings where you can connect with individuals who have gone through similar experiences. Engaging in positive interactions and fostering meaningful connections with supportive people nourishes your emotional and social well-being, contributing to overall self-care and personal growth.

In summary, connecting with supportive people is essential for caring for yourself physically, mentally, emotionally, and spiritually after leaving a toxic relationship. Identify supportive individuals and groups who can provide understanding and validation. Communicate your needs and boundaries to your support network to receive the specific support you require. Actively engage in activities and shared experiences to foster a sense of belonging and connection. By surrounding yourself with supportive people, you create an environment that nurtures your well-being and empowers you on your healing journey.

12 Steps to Recovering from A Toxic Relationship

Set boundaries.

Setting boundaries is crucial for caring for yourself holistically after getting out of a toxic relationship. Firstly, take the time to reflect on your needs and values. Next, identify what is important to you and what you are comfortable with. This self-awareness will guide you in establishing clear and firm boundaries. Finally, recognize that setting boundaries is an act of self-care and self-respect, allowing you to protect your physical, mental, emotional, and spiritual well-being.

Secondly, communicate your boundaries assertively and effectively. Clearly express your limits, expectations, and what you will no longer tolerate. Use "I" statements to convey your needs and feelings, focusing on expressing yourself without blaming or criticizing others. Be firm and consistent in maintaining your boundaries, even if it may initially be met with resistance. Remember that your boundaries are valid and essential for your overall well-being.

Lastly, be prepared to enforce your boundaries. This may involve saying no to activities, conversations, or behaviors that cross your boundaries. It's important to prioritize your well-being and not feel guilty for prioritizing yourself. Surround yourself with supportive people who respect your boundaries and distance yourself from those who consistently disregard them. By setting and enforcing boundaries, you create a safe and nurturing environment that allows you to care for yourself holistically.

Setting boundaries is crucial to caring for yourself physically, mentally, emotionally, and spiritually after leaving a toxic relationship. Reflect on your needs and values to determine the necessary boundaries for your well-being. Communicate your boundaries assertively and effectively, expressing your needs without blaming or criticizing others. Be prepared to enforce your boundaries and surround yourself with supportive individuals who respect and honor them. Setting boundaries is an empowering act of self-care that enables you to prioritize your well-being and create a healthier and more fulfilling life.

Pursue your passions.

Pursuing your passions is a powerful way to care for yourself holistically after getting out of a toxic relationship. Firstly, take the time to rediscover your interests and hobbies. Then, reflect on the activities that bring you joy, ignite your creativity, or provide a sense of fulfillment. This could be anything from painting, writing, playing an instrument, practicing yoga, or engaging in outdoor activities. By actively pursuing your passions, you tap into a source of self-expression and personal fulfillment, contributing to your overall well-being.

Secondly, make space in your life to dedicate time and energy to your passions. Prioritize your needs and allocate specific time slots for engaging in activities that bring you joy and fulfillment. This may involve setting boundaries with others and creating a routine that supports the pursuit of your passions. Nurturing that investing in yourself and nurturing your interests is not selfish but rather an essential part of self-care. Dedicating time to your passions creates a sense of purpose, self-discovery, and personal growth that positively impacts your physical, mental, emotional, and spiritual well-being.

Lastly, seek opportunities to connect with like-minded individuals who share your passions. Join clubs, organizations, or communities centered around your interests. Engaging with others who have similar passions creates a sense of belonging, provides support, and fosters new friendships. Sharing your experiences, ideas, and achievements with others who appreciate and understand your passions enhances your well-being. It allows you to cultivate a supportive network that nourishes your physical, mental, emotional, and spiritual health.

In summary, pursuing your passions is a powerful way to care for yourself holistically after leaving a toxic relationship. Rediscover your interests and hobbies, making them a priority in your life. Dedicate time and energy to engage in activities that bring you joy and fulfillment. Seek opportunities to connect with like-minded individuals who share your passions. By pursuing your passions, you cultivate a sense of purpose, self-expression, and personal growth that contributes to your overall well-being and helps you navigate your healing journey.

Practice mindfulness.

Practicing mindfulness is a powerful way to care for yourself holistically after getting out of a toxic relationship. Firstly, cultivate awareness of the present moment. Pay attention to your thoughts, emotions, and sensations without judgment or attachment. Acknowledge and accept your experiences as they arise, allowing yourself to process and understand your feelings fully. Mindfulness helps you stay grounded in the present, fostering a sense of calm and stability amidst challenging emotions or situations.

Secondly, incorporate mindfulness into your daily routine. Set aside time for mindfulness practices such as meditation, deep breathing exercises, or body scans. These practices allow you to connect with yourself, release tension, and cultivate inner peace. Additionally, bring mindfulness into your daily activities by paying attention to your senses, engaging fully in each task, and savoring the present moment. Mindful eating, walking, or engaging in any activity with full awareness helps to anchor you in the present and promotes self-care across all dimensions of your well-being.

Lastly, use mindfulness to develop self-compassion and cultivate a loving and accepting relationship with yourself. Offer kindness, understanding, and forgiveness as you navigate the healing process. Notice any self-judgment or self-critical thoughts and gently redirect your attention to self-compassion. Treat yourself with the same kindness and care you would

12 Steps to Recovering from A Toxic Relationship

extend to a loved one. Mindfulness allows you to tune into your needs, practice self-care, and nurture yourself physically, mentally, emotionally, and spiritually.

Practicing mindfulness is a transformative way to care for yourself holistically after leaving a toxic relationship. Cultivate awareness of the present moment, allowing yourself to experience and process your thoughts and emotions fully. Incorporate mindfulness into your daily routine through dedicated practices and mindful engagement in daily activities. Use mindfulness to develop self-compassion and cultivate a loving relationship with yourself. Practicing mindfulness fosters a sense of inner peace, resilience, and self-care that supports your overall well-being and helps you navigate your healing journey.

Get creative.

Getting creative is a wonderful way to care for yourself holistically after getting out of a toxic relationship. Firstly, tap into your imagination and explore different forms of artistic expression. Engage in painting, drawing, writing, dancing, or playing a musical instrument. Allow yourself the freedom to express your emotions, thoughts, and experiences through these creative outlets. Creating can be cathartic, allowing you to process and release any pent-up emotions while providing a channel for self-expression and self-discovery.

Secondly, embrace experimentation and try new things. Step outside your comfort zone and explore creative endeavors you've always been curious about but never had the chance to pursue. Take a cooking class, learn a new craft, or explore photography. Engaging in new creative experiences stimulates your mind, ignites your curiosity, and opens you up to new possibilities. This process of exploration and discovery enhances your mental and emotional well-being, expands your horizons, and brings a sense of joy and fulfillment.

Lastly, seek inspiration from others and engage in collaborative creative projects. Connect with like-minded individuals who share your passion for creativity and collaborate on artistic ventures. Join art communities, attend workshops, or participate in group projects. Collaborating with others fosters a sense of belonging and community and provides a space for shared learning and growth. In addition, by engaging in collaborative creative endeavors, you tap into the collective energy, creativity, and support of others, nurturing your emotional and spiritual well-being.

In summary, getting creative is a powerful way to care for yourself physically, mentally, emotionally, and spiritually after leaving a toxic relationship. Tap into your imagination and express yourself through various artistic forms. Embrace experimentation and try new creative endeavors that spark your curiosity. Seek inspiration from others and engage in collaborative projects to foster a sense of connection and shared growth. By getting creative, you encourage self-expression, self-discovery, and a sense of joy that contributes to your overall well-being and helps you cultivate a fulfilling and meaningful life after a toxic relationship.

Connect with your spiritual side.

Connecting with your spiritual side is a powerful way to care for yourself holistically after getting out of a toxic relationship. Firstly, take time for self-reflection and introspection. Then, set aside moments of quiet and solitude to connect with your inner self and explore your beliefs, values, and purpose. Next, meditate, journal, or pray to deepen your connection with your spirituality. These practices help you find inner peace, clarity, and purpose, allowing you to navigate your healing journey with a solid foundation.

Secondly, explore different spiritual traditions and teachings. Attend spiritual gatherings, workshops, or retreats that align with your interests. Engage in conversations with individuals who share similar spiritual beliefs and seek out mentors or guides who can provide guidance and support. By immersing yourself in spiritual practices, you expand your understanding of spirituality and find solace in a community that shares your beliefs and values. This connection with your spiritual side nurtures your emotional well-being and provides comfort and strength.

Lastly, integrate your spirituality into your daily life. Find ways to infuse spiritual practices into your routines and activities. This can include incorporating mindfulness into your daily tasks, expressing gratitude for blessings, or engaging in acts of service and kindness toward others. By weaving spirituality into your everyday experiences, you create a more profound sense of meaning, fulfillment, and connection with the world around you. This connection with your spiritual side supports your overall well-being and helps you find balance and resilience as you move forward from the toxic relationship.

In summary, connecting with your spiritual side is a transformative way to care for yourself physically, mentally, emotionally, and spiritually after leaving a toxic relationship. Engage in self-reflection and introspection to deepen your connection with your inner self. Explore different spiritual traditions and teachings to expand your understanding of spirituality and find support within a like-minded community. Integrate your spirituality into daily life by infusing spiritual practices into your routines and activities. By nurturing your spiritual well-being, you cultivate a sense of purpose, inner peace, and connection that supports your overall well-being and helps you thrive after a toxic relationship. Caring for oneself after a toxic breakup is crucial to the healing process. It's important to prioritize self-care in all areas of life, including physical, mental, emotional, and spiritual health. Physically, this could mean exercising regularly, eating a healthy diet, and getting enough sleep. Taking care of basic physical needs can help support mental and emotional well-being. Emotionally, practicing self-compassion, managing stress, and seeking support from loved ones or a therapist is essential. Acknowledging and processing emotions that arise after a toxic breakup can help a person move forward positively.

Mentally, practicing mindfulness and pursuing creative outlets can help a person stay present at the moment and healthily process their emotions. Finally, connecting with one's spirituality through prayer or meditation can help one find purpose and meaning after a toxic breakup. By taking the time to care for oneself in these ways, a person can rebuild their sense of self-worth and set the stage for a brighter, healthier future filled with opportunities for growth, self-discovery, and happiness.

Step 11: Practice Self-Kindness. "Speak Life into Yourself."

Self-kindness is an essential component of self-care that involves treating oneself with kindness, understanding, and compassion. It is about being gentle with oneself and prioritizing one's emotional and mental well-being. Many people struggle with self-criticism and negative self-talk, which can affect their mental health. Practicing self-kindness can help individuals build a stronger sense of self-worth, improve their mood, and reduce stress and anxiety. In addition, individuals can cultivate a more positive mindset and a greater understanding of self-love by caring for themselves with kindness and compassion. In this way, practicing self-kindness is integral to achieving overall well-being.

Practice self-compassion.

Practicing self-compassion and speaking life into yourself is a powerful way to cultivate self-kindness and promote healing after getting out of a toxic relationship. Firstly, become aware of your self-talk and challenge negative or self-critical thoughts. Replace them with positive affirmations and words of encouragement. Remind yourself of your strengths, resilience, and worthiness. Speak to yourself as you would to a dear friend, offering compassion, understanding, and support. By practicing positive self-

12 Steps to Recovering from A Toxic Relationship

talk, you shift your mindset towards self-acceptance and self-love.

Secondly, prioritize self-care and engage in activities that nourish your body, mind, and soul. Set aside time daily for self-care rituals that bring you joy and relaxation. This can include practicing mindfulness, engaging in physical exercise, enjoying a soothing bath, or indulging in hobbies that please you. By intentionally caring for yourself, you send a powerful message of self-worth and prioritize your well-being. These acts of self-care foster a sense of self-compassion and reinforce the belief that you deserve kindness and happiness.

Lastly, practice forgiveness towards yourself for any perceived shortcomings or mistakes. Acknowledge that you are human and that everyone makes errors. Release the burden of guilt or shame and offer yourself forgiveness and understanding. Embrace a growth mindset and view challenges as opportunities for growth and learning. By practicing self-forgiveness, you let go of self-judgment and open yourself up to personal growth and transformation.

In summary, practicing self-compassion and speaking life into yourself is a transformative way to practice self-kindness after leaving a toxic relationship. Challenge negative self-talk and replace it with positive affirmations and words of encouragement. Prioritize self-care and engage in activities that nourish your well-being. Practice forgiveness towards yourself and embrace a growth mindset. By cultivating self-compassion, you foster self-acceptance, resilience, and personal growth as you move forward on your journey of healing and self-discovery.

Take time for yourself.

Taking time for yourself is an essential practice of self-kindness and speaking life into yourself after getting out of a toxic relationship. Firstly, carve out moments of solitude and reflection to reconnect with your inner self. Next, create a daily routine that includes dedicated time for self-care, whether it's a quiet walk-in nature, reading a book that inspires you, or simply enjoying a cup of tea while practicing mindfulness. These moments of solitude allow you to recharge, listen to your inner voice, and honor your needs and desires.

Secondly, set boundaries and protect your personal space and time. Learn to say no to activities or commitments that do not align with your well-being or values. Prioritize yourself by establishing clear boundaries with others and communicating your needs effectively. This may involve setting limits on social interactions, taking breaks from technology or social media, or creating designated "me-time" where you can engage in activities that bring you joy and peace. You reinforce the importance of self-kindness and self-care by respecting your boundaries and honoring your time.

Lastly, explore activities that bring you happiness and fulfillment. Engage in hobbies or passions that ignite your creativity and allow you to express yourself authentically. Whether painting, dancing, writing, or playing an instrument, immerse yourself in activities that bring joy and a sense of purpose. By dedicating time to these activities, you honor your passions and nurture your well-being, allowing yourself to thrive and grow.

In summary, taking time for yourself is a crucial practice of self-kindness and speaking life into yourself after leaving a toxic relationship. Create moments of solitude and reflection to reconnect with your inner self and honor your needs. Set boundaries to protect your personal space and time and prioritize self-care. Engage in activities that bring you happiness and fulfillment, allowing you to explore and express your authentic self. By prioritizing yourself and dedicating time to self-care, you cultivate a strong foundation of self-kindness, love, and empowerment as you navigate your healing journey.

Set healthy boundaries.

Setting healthy boundaries is important to practicing self-kindness and speaking life into yourself after getting out of a toxic relationship. Firstly, recognize and honor your own needs and values. Then, take the time to reflect on what is important to you and what makes you feel comfortable and safe. Finally, understanding your boundaries allows you to communicate them to others, ensuring your needs and well-being are respected.

Secondly, learn to say no without guilt or apology. It is essential to set limits and prioritize your well-being. Saying no to situations, people, or requests that do not align with your boundaries is an act of self-care and self-preservation. Trust yourself and your instincts when deciding what feels right for you. Remember that setting boundaries is not selfish but a way to protect your mental, emotional, and physical health.

Lastly, communicate your boundaries effectively and assertively. Clearly express your limits and expectations to others, using "I" statements to convey your feelings and needs. Be firm yet respectful in your communication, understanding that you can advocate for yourself and set boundaries that support your well-being. Surround yourself with individuals who respect and honor your boundaries, and distance yourself from those who consistently disregard them. You create an environment that promotes self-kindness, self-respect, and personal growth by setting healthy boundaries.

In summary, setting healthy boundaries is an act of self-kindness and speaking life into yourself after leaving a toxic relationship. Understand and honor your needs and values, learning to say no without guilt or apology. Communicate your boundaries effectively and assertively, advocating for your well-being. Surround yourself with individuals who respect your boundaries and distance yourself from those who do not. By setting healthy boundaries, you create a space that fosters self-care, self-compassion, and personal growth as you navigate your healing journey.

Engage in positive self-talk.

Positive self-talk is a powerful practice of self-kindness and speaking life into yourself after getting out of a toxic relationship. Firstly, become aware of your inner dialogue and the thoughts you consistently have about yourself. Then, notice any negative or self-critical thoughts that arise and consciously replace them with positive affirmations and supportive statements. For example, when you think, "I'm not good enough," reframe it into, "I am worthy and deserving of love and happiness."

Secondly, practice self-compassion by treating yourself with kindness, understanding, and acceptance. Be gentle with yourself and acknowledge that healing takes time. Instead of beating yourself up over past mistakes or dwelling on perceived shortcomings, focus on your progress and growth. Celebrate your achievements, no matter how small, and remind yourself of your strengths and resilience. Embrace a mindset of self-love and self-acceptance, nurturing a positive relationship with yourself.

Lastly, surround yourself with positive influences and affirmations. Seek inspirational books, podcasts, or quotes that uplift and motivate you. Write down positive affirmations that resonate with you and repeat them daily. Create a supportive environment by surrounding yourself with people who encourage and believe in you. Positive self-talk is not about denying reality or avoiding challenges but cultivating a mindset that empowers and motivates you to overcome obstacles and embrace your worth.

In summary, positive self-talk is a powerful practice of self-kindness and speaking life into yourself after leaving a toxic relationship. Become aware of your inner dialogue and consciously replace negative thoughts with positive affirmations. Practice self-compassion and celebrate your progress and growth. Surround yourself with positive influences and affirmations, creating a supportive environment that nurtures self-love and empowers you to embrace your worth. Through positive self-talk, you cultivate a mindset of self-kindness, resilience, and empowerment as you navigate your healing journey.

Cultivate a positive mindset:

Cultivating a positive mindset is a powerful way to practice self-kindness and speak life into yourself after getting out of a toxic relationship. Firstly, focus on gratitude and count your blessings. Then, take time each day to reflect on the things you are grateful for, no matter how small they may seem. This practice shifts your perspective towards positivity and reminds you of the good things in your life. By cultivating gratitude, you invite positivity and appreciation into your daily experiences.

Secondly, challenge negative thoughts and replace them with positive affirmations. Notice when negative self-talk arises and consciously choose to reframe those thoughts. For example, if you think, "I'll never find love again," counteract it with a positive affirmation like, "I am deserving of love, and I trust that the right person will come into my life at the right time." By consciously choosing positive thoughts, you rewire your mindset and create a foundation of self-belief and optimism.

Lastly, surround yourself with positivity. Engage in activities, hobbies, and relationships that uplift and inspire you. Seek out positive and motivational resources like books, podcasts, or inspirational quotes that resonate with you. Surround yourself with supportive and encouraging people who believe in your potential and help you see the best in yourself. By cultivating a positive environment and mindset, you create a nurturing space for self-kindness, self-empowerment, and personal growth.

In summary, cultivating a positive mindset is a powerful practice of self-kindness and speaking life into yourself after leaving a toxic relationship. Focus on gratitude and count your blessings to shift your perspective towards positivity. Next, challenge negative thoughts and replace them with positive affirmations reinforcing your self-worth and belief in yourself. Finally, surround yourself with positivity through activities, resources, and relationships that uplift and inspire you. By cultivating a positive mindset, you foster self-kindness, resilience, and an empowered outlook as you continue your healing journey.

Practice forgiveness.

Practicing forgiveness is a powerful way to practice self-kindness and speak life into yourself after getting out of a toxic relationship. Firstly, recognize that forgiveness is not about condoning or excusing the harmful actions of others but rather about releasing the negative emotions and burdens that come with holding onto grudges. By forgiving, you free yourself from the weight of anger, resentment, and bitterness, allowing space for healing and personal growth.

Secondly, extend forgiveness to yourself. Understand that you are human and may have made mistakes or had moments of vulnerability during the toxic relationship. Instead of blaming yourself or holding onto self-judgment, practice self-compassion and forgive yourself. Recognize that you deserve understanding, love, and acceptance, as anyone else does. Release self-criticism and embrace self-forgiveness to cultivate self-kindness and nurture your emotional well-being.

Lastly, focus on the future rather than dwelling on the past. Forgiveness lets you let go of past hurts and create space for new experiences and opportunities. By shifting your focus to the present moment and envisioning a positive future, you release the negative energy that may have been holding you back. Practice self-kindness by setting realistic goals, pursuing your passions, and surrounding yourself with supportive people who uplift and inspire you. Embrace forgiveness as a personal growth and self-empowerment tool, allowing yourself to thrive beyond toxic relationships.

In summary, practicing forgiveness is a transformative practice of self-kindness and speaking life into yourself after leaving a toxic relationship. Extend forgiveness to others, releasing the negative emotions and burdens of holding onto grudges. Offer yourself forgiveness, recognize your humanity, and embrace self-compassion. Focus on the future and create a positive vision, setting realistic goals and surrounding yourself with supportive people. Through forgiveness, you cultivate self-kindness, emotional healing, and a renewed sense of empowerment as you continue to embrace your journey of self-discovery and personal happiness.

Engage in activities that promote relaxation.

Engaging in activities that promote relaxation is an essential way to practice self-kindness and speak life into yourself after getting out of a toxic relationship. Firstly, prioritize self-care and make it a part of your daily routine. Next, take time for activities that bring you peace and relaxation, such as practicing mindfulness, soothing baths, or enjoying nature walks. These activities allow you to unwind, reduce stress, and nurture your well-being.

Secondly, explore different relaxation techniques and find what works best for you. This could include deep breathing exercises, meditation, yoga, or listening to calming music. Again, experiment with various techniques and observe how each makes you feel. Regularly engaging in these practices creates a space for self-kindness and inner peace, allowing you to recharge and rejuvenate.

Lastly, disconnect from technology and create sacred spaces for relaxation. In our fast-paced, digitally connected world, carving out time to unplug and be present with yourself is important. Designate certain areas in your home as relaxation spaces, free from distractions and noise. This could be a cozy corner with comfortable cushions, a calming room with soft lighting, or an outdoor sanctuary surrounded by nature. You create an environment conducive to self-kindness, introspection, and relaxation by intentionally creating these spaces and disconnecting from the outside world.

In summary, engaging in activities that promote relaxation is a powerful practice of self-kindness and speaking life into yourself after leaving a toxic relationship. Prioritize self-care and incorporate relaxation activities into your daily routine. Explore different relaxation techniques and find what resonates with you. Disconnect from technology and create sacred spaces where you can unwind and be present with yourself. These activities create a nurturing environment for self-kindness, inner peace, and emotional well-being as you continue to heal and rediscover your happiness.

12 Steps to Recovering from A Toxic Relationship

Celebrate your accomplishments.

Celebrating your accomplishments is a powerful way to practice self-kindness and speak life into yourself after getting out of a toxic relationship. Firstly, acknowledge and appreciate your achievements, no matter how small they may seem. Next, recognize that overcoming the challenges of a toxic relationship takes strength, resilience, and courage. Finally, take on your progress and credit yourself for your steps toward healing and personal growth.

Secondly, create a ritual of celebration for your accomplishments. This could involve treating yourself to something special, such as a relaxing spa day, a favorite meal, or a day trip to a place you love. Celebrate your achievements in a way that feels meaningful and uplifting to you. By consciously honoring your milestones, you reinforce a positive mindset and self-worth, reminding yourself that you deserve love, happiness, and success.

Lastly, share your accomplishments with supportive people in your life. Surround yourself with individuals who genuinely celebrate your wins and uplift you. For example, share your progress with trusted friends or family members who can offer encouragement and validation. By sharing your accomplishments, you invite positive energy and affirmations into your life, boosting your self-esteem and reinforcing your belief in your capabilities.

In summary, celebrating your accomplishments is a powerful practice of self-kindness and speaking life into yourself after leaving a toxic relationship. Acknowledge and appreciate your achievements, no matter how small. Create rituals of celebration that honor your progress and make you feel special. Share your accomplishments with supportive people who celebrate your wins. By embracing this practice, you nurture self-kindness, foster a positive self-image, and empower yourself to continue healing and personal transformation.

Practice self-care.

Practicing self-care is essential to practicing self-kindness and speaking life into yourself after getting out of a toxic relationship. Firstly, prioritize your physical well-being by taking care of your body. This can include getting enough sleep, eating nutritious meals, and exercising regularly. Nourishing your body with healthy habits allows you to cultivate self-kindness, show yourself the love, and care you deserve.

Secondly, tend to your emotional and mental well-being by engaging in activities that bring you joy and peace. This can involve practicing mindfulness and meditation, journaling your thoughts and feelings, or engaging in creative outlets such as painting, writing, or playing music. Taking time for these activities allows you to connect with yourself deeper, process your emotions, and practice self-compassion.

Lastly, set boundaries and protect your energy by saying no to things that drain you and yes to things that uplift and inspire you. This includes prioritizing self-care activities that rejuvenate your spirit, such as taking long baths, enjoying nature walks, or engaging in hobbies that bring you joy. By intentionally carving out time for self-care, you send a powerful message to yourself that your well-being matters and that you are worthy of love, care, and kindness.

In summary, practicing self-care is a transformative practice of self-kindness and speaking life into yourself after leaving a toxic relationship. Prioritize your physical well-being, engage in activities that nourish your emotional and mental health, and set boundaries to protect your energy. By actively practicing self-care, you honor your worth, cultivate self-compassion, and create a foundation of self-kindness that supports your healing journey and allows you to embrace a life filled with love, happiness, and fulfillment.

Surround yourself with positive people.

Surrounding yourself with positive people is a powerful way to practice self-kindness and speak life into yourself after getting out of a toxic relationship. Firstly, identify the individuals who radiate positivity, support, and genuine care. These people uplift you, inspire you, and believe in your worth. Then, prioritize spending time with them and nurturing those relationships.

Secondly, create a supportive network by seeking like-minded individuals with similar values and interests. This can be done through joining clubs, organizations, or communities centered around hobbies, passions, or causes that resonate with you. Engaging with positive people who share common goals and aspirations can give you a sense of belonging, support, and encouragement.

Lastly, practice setting boundaries with toxic or negative individuals. Surrounding yourself with positive people also means removing or minimizing contact with those who drain your energy or bring negativity into your life. It's important to prioritize your well-being and protect yourself from toxic influences. Surrounding yourself with positive people who uplift and inspire you creates an environment of support and kindness, enabling you to speak life into yourself and cultivate self-kindness.

In summary, surrounding yourself with positive people is a powerful practice of self-kindness and speaking life into yourself after leaving a toxic relationship. Identify and prioritize relationships with individuals who radiate positivity and support. Seek out like-minded individuals through shared interests and values. Set boundaries with toxic individuals to protect your well-being. By cultivating a network of positive people, you create a supportive environment that fosters self-kindness, boosts your self-esteem, and empowers you to continue your healing and personal growth journey.

12 Steps to Recovering from A Toxic Relationship

Practicing self-kindness and speaking life into yourself is crucial for personal growth, well-being, and happiness. Firstly, practicing self-kindness allows you to cultivate a healthy and positive relationship with yourself. It involves treating yourself with compassion, understanding, and acceptance, regardless of past experiences or mistakes. By practicing self-kindness, you learn to nurture and care for your needs, boosting your self-esteem and self-worth.

Secondly, speaking life into yourself through positive self-talk and affirmations helps to reframe negative thoughts and beliefs. It involves replacing self-criticism with self-encouragement, self-acceptance, and self-love. By consciously choosing empowering and uplifting words, you can change how you perceive yourself and your capabilities. This shift in mindset opens up new possibilities, builds resilience, and fosters a sense of inner strength and confidence.

Lastly, practicing self-kindness and speaking life into yourself promotes overall well-being. It allows you to prioritize self-care and engage in activities that nourish your mind, body, and soul. Honoring your needs and boundaries creates a healthy balance in your life, reduces stress, and improves your overall happiness and satisfaction. Self-kindness also enhances your relationships with others, as you can show up authentically and offer genuine care and support when taking care of yourself first.

In summary, practicing self-kindness and speaking life into yourself is a transformative practice that benefits every aspect of your life. It fosters self-acceptance, builds resilience, and nurtures a positive mindset. You create a foundation for personal growth, happiness, and fulfilling relationships by valuing and caring for yourself. Embracing self-kindness is a lifelong journey that empowers you to live authentically, celebrate your strengths, and embrace your unique worthiness.

12 Steps to Recovering from A Toxic Relationship

"Speak Life Into Yourself" Quotes:

"Many people, especially ignorant people, want to punish you for speaking the truth, being correct, and being you. Never apologize for being correct or for being years ahead of your time. If you're right and you know it, speak your mind. Speak your mind. Even if you are a minority of one, the truth is still the truth."

-Mahatma Gandhi

"It's better to speak your mind and tell the truth than to stay quiet and lie to yourself."
-Anonymous

Step 12: Don't Check In On Your Ex Once Out Of Your Negative Situation

After a toxic breakup, the urge to check in on an ex can be overwhelming and hard to resist. Whether out of loneliness, curiosity, or a desire for closure, checking in on an ex can reignite old wounds and make it difficult to move on. While it is normal to have these urges, individuals need to resist the temptation to check in on their ex and focus on their healing and growth. By taking proactive steps to avoid checking in, individuals can establish healthy boundaries, protect their emotional well-being, and create space for personal development. In this prompt, we will explore ten concrete strategies individuals can use to resist checking in on their ex after a toxic breakup. These strategies range from practical steps like deleting contact information and setting boundaries to emotional coping strategies like journaling and seeking professional help. With the right mindset and tools, individuals can break the cycle of checking in on their ex and move forward with confidence and self-assurance.

Delete their contact information and unfollow them on social media.

Deleting your ex's contact information and unfollowing them on social media after ending a negative relationship can be essential to your healing and growth. Firstly, it allows you to create healthy boundaries and protect yourself from further emotional turmoil. Checking in on your ex or keeping tabs on their life through social media can lead to feelings of jealousy, sadness, or even anger, which hinders your progress in moving on. By deleting their contact information and unfollowing it, you free yourself from the constant reminders and triggers that may hold you back from finding peace and happiness.

Secondly, it enables you to reclaim your identity and focus on your journey of self-discovery. After ending a toxic relationship, shifting the focus back to yourself and prioritizing your well-being is crucial. Constantly checking on your ex's social media updates or maintaining contact can prevent you from fully detaching and moving forward. Instead, removing this connection creates space for personal growth, self-reflection, and the opportunity to rebuild your life on your terms.

Lastly, deleting their contact information and unfollowing them allows you to break free from any potential cycles of toxicity or negativity. It signifies your commitment to creating a healthier and happier future for yourself. Cutting off contact removes the potential for further emotional manipulation or hurtful interactions. It empowers you to choose your path and surround yourself with positivity, allowing you to focus on cultivating healthy relationships and a more fulfilling life.

In conclusion, deleting your ex's contact information and unfollowing them on social media is crucial to your healing, growth, and happiness after ending a negative relationship. It helps establish healthy boundaries, enables you to focus on your journey of self-discovery, and breaks free from potential cycles of toxicity. In addition, by taking this action, you create the space needed to fully detach and move forward, paving the way for a brighter and more fulfilling future.

Replace the urge to check in with a different activity, such as exercise or a hobby.

Replacing the urge to check in on your ex with a different activity, such as exercise or a hobby, is crucial for your emotional well-being and growth after ending a negative relationship. Firstly, it helps to break the cycle of constant thoughts and preoccupation with your ex. You redirect your attention and energy towards something positive and fulfilling by engaging in physical activity or pursuing a hobby. This shift in focus allows you to regain control over your thoughts and emotions, reducing the chances of getting trapped in a cycle of rumination and overthinking about your past relationship.

Secondly, engaging in a different activity provides an opportunity for self-care and self-discovery. Exercise, for example, has numerous physical and mental health benefits. It releases endorphins, improves mood, and reduces stress levels. By prioritizing your well-being through activities like exercise or hobbies, you reinforce the importance of self-care and self-compassion. It allows you to reconnect with yourself, your passions, and your personal growth, fostering a sense of empowerment and independence.

Lastly, replacing the urge to check in with a different activity creates space for healing and moving forward. Continually checking in on your ex can keep you emotionally attached and hinder your ability to let go of the past entirely. Engaging in a new activity helps you create new experiences, form new connections, and develop a sense of identity outside the relationship. It allows you to redefine yourself and your future, free from the emotional baggage of the past. Focusing on your growth and well-being creates a solid foundation for building a healthier and happier life.

In conclusion, replacing the urge to check in on your ex with a different activity, such as exercise or a hobby, is essential for your emotional healing and personal growth after leaving a negative relationship. It breaks the cycle of constant thoughts, promotes self-care and self-discovery, and creates space for healing and moving forward. By redirecting your energy towards positive and fulfilling activities, you regain control over your thoughts and emotions, prioritize your well-being, and open the door to new experiences and a brighter future.

Reach out to supportive friends or family members for distraction and encouragement.

Reaching out to supportive friends or family members for distraction and encouragement is crucial when you're tempted to check on your ex after ending a negative relationship. Firstly, these individuals can provide a much-needed distraction from the thoughts and emotions surrounding your past relationship. Engaging in meaningful conversations or activities with supportive friends or family shifts your focus away from your ex and towards positive interactions and experiences. Their presence can help redirect your attention and remind you of the importance of nurturing healthy relationships.

Secondly, supportive friends and family members can offer encouragement and validation during this challenging time. They can provide a listening ear, empathy, and understanding as you navigate moving on. Their reassurance and perspective can help you gain clarity and remind you of your worth outside the toxic relationship. By seeking their support, you create a support system that uplifts and empowers you, promoting emotional well-being and resilience.

Lastly, reaching out to supportive friends or family fosters a sense of connection and belonging. Surrounding yourself with individuals who genuinely care for your well-being and want to see you thrive can profoundly impact your mental and emotional state. It helps combat feelings of loneliness and isolation that often arise after a negative relationship ends. By leaning on your support network, you create an environment of positivity and growth, strengthening your ability to move forward and build a happier and healthier future.

In conclusion, reaching out to supportive friends or family members for distraction and encouragement is essential when you're tempted to check on your ex after leaving a negative relationship. Their presence provides a valuable distraction from the past, offers encouragement and validation, and promotes a sense of connection and belonging. In addition, by seeking their support, you surround yourself with a supportive network that uplifts and empowers you, helping you navigate the healing process and embrace a brighter future.

Journal about feelings of loneliness or sadness instead of acting on the urge to check in.

Journaling about feelings of loneliness or sadness instead of acting on the urge to check on your ex can be incredibly beneficial for your emotional well-being and personal growth. Firstly, journaling provides a safe and private space to express and process emotions. It allows you to freely explore your thoughts, feelings, and experiences without judgment or interruption. Finally, putting pen to paper will enable you to release pent-up emotions and gain clarity about your emotional state.

Secondly, journaling helps you gain insight into your patterns and triggers. By regularly documenting your feelings of loneliness or sadness, you can start to identify common themes or situations that trigger these emotions. This self-awareness is crucial for personal growth and healing. It allows you to recognize any underlying patterns or unresolved issues that need attention, helping you to break free from negative cycles and make positive changes in your life.

Lastly, journaling can provide a sense of empowerment and control. You take ownership of your emotional well-being when you write about your feelings rather than engaging in impulsive behaviors like checking on your ex. It allows you to process your emotions and constructively work through them actively. By reflecting and writing, you regain control over your thoughts and actions, empowering yourself to make healthier choices that support your overall well-being.

In conclusion, journaling about feelings of loneliness or sadness instead of acting on the urge to check on your ex is a powerful tool for emotional healing and personal growth. It provides a safe space to express and process your emotions, helps you gain insight into your patterns and triggers, and empowers you to take control of your emotional well-being. By making journaling a regular practice, you can navigate the healing process more effectively and cultivate a deeper understanding of yourself, leading to greater self-compassion.

12 Steps to Recovering from A Toxic Relationship

Remind yourself of the reasons why the relationship was toxic and why it is vital to move on.

Reminding yourself of why the relationship was toxic and why it is vital to move on instead of checking on your ex is essential for your healing and growth. Firstly, reflecting on the relationship's toxic aspects helps you reaffirm your decision to end it. By recalling the negative patterns, behaviors, and dynamics present, you reinforce that staying connected to your ex would only perpetuate the toxicity and hinder your progress toward a healthier and happier life.

Secondly, reminding yourself of the toxic elements helps you to maintain perspective and stay focused on your well-being. It serves as a reality check and prevents you from romanticizing the past or idealizing your ex. By keeping in mind the harmful dynamics that existed, you are less likely to get trapped in a cycle of longing or nostalgia. This allows you to prioritize your happiness and make choices that align with your self-respect and growth.

Lastly, reminding yourself of the toxicity in the relationship is a form of self-protection and self-care. It protects against potential emotional harm or relapse into negative patterns. By consciously choosing to let go and move on, you create space for healing, personal growth, and healthier relationships in the future. It empowers you to break free from the grip of the past and create a new narrative for yourself—one that is rooted in self-love, respect, and positive experiences.

In conclusion, reminding yourself why the relationship was toxic and moving on instead of checking on your ex is crucial for your healing and well-being. It strengthens your resolve to avoid a toxic situation, maintains perspective, and protects you from potential emotional harm. Focusing on your growth and happiness creates the space for a brighter future and healthier relationships. Embracing this mindset allows you to break free from the past and embrace the possibilities that lie ahead.

Seek professional help or counseling to process difficult emotions and thoughts.

Seeking professional help or counseling to process difficult emotions and thoughts instead of checking on your ex is a wise decision that can significantly aid your healing and growth. Firstly, a trained therapist or counselor provides a safe and non-judgmental space to express and explore your feelings related to the past relationship. They can help you gain insight into the dynamics of toxic relationships, identify patterns, and work through any unresolved emotional baggage.

Secondly, professional help can provide valuable tools and strategies to cope with the challenges arising from a toxic relationship's end. They can assist you in developing healthy coping mechanisms, building resilience, and managing stress and anxiety. By equipping you with these skills, therapy or counseling empowers you to navigate the complexities of your emotions and thoughts constructively and productively.

Lastly, seeking professional help fosters personal growth and self-discovery. A skilled therapist or counselor can guide you in exploring your values, beliefs, and goals. They can help you redefine your identity, rebuild your self-esteem, and set healthy boundaries in future relationships. Working with a professional can facilitate a transformative journey toward self-empowerment, self-compassion, and personal fulfillment.

In summary, seeking professional help or counseling to process difficult emotions and thoughts instead of checking on your ex offers numerous benefits. It provides a professional environment to process your experiences, equips you with effective coping strategies, and facilitates personal growth and self-discovery. In addition, therapy or counseling can be instrumental in your healing journey, helping you move forward.

Create a daily self-care routine that includes activities that bring you joy and fulfillment.

Creating a daily self-care routine that prioritizes activities bringing you joy and fulfillment is essential after getting out of a negative relationship, instead of constantly checking on your ex. Firstly, self-care allows you to redirect your energy and focus on your well-being. It provides a nurturing space to recharge, rejuvenate, and reconnect with yourself. By consciously investing time and effort into activities that bring you joy and fulfillment, you reinforce a positive and loving relationship with yourself, which is vital for healing and personal growth.

Secondly, a self-care routine helps to shift your attention away from the past and onto the present moment. Engaging in activities that bring you joy, whether practicing a hobby, spending time in nature, or enjoying a creative outlet, promotes a sense of presence and mindfulness. By immersing yourself in activities that bring you fulfillment, you cultivate a deeper connection with yourself and the world around you, fostering a positive mindset and reducing the temptation to dwell on the past or check on your ex.

Lastly, incorporating self-care activities into your daily routine fosters self-compassion and self-acceptance. It sends a powerful message that you deserve love, care, and happiness. You prioritize your well-being and demonstrate self-compassion by intentionally engaging in activities that bring you joy and fulfillment. This practice helps build a strong foundation of self-worth, reminding you that you deserve happiness and fulfillment independent of your past relationships.

In summary, creating a daily self-care routine that includes activities bringing you joy and fulfillment is crucial after getting out of a negative relationship. It allows you to focus on your well-being, shift your attention to the present moment, and cultivate self-compassion. In addition, by engaging in activities that bring you joy, you nourish your mind, body, and soul, helping you heal, grow, and move forward in a positive and fulfilling way.

Use positive affirmations or mantras to shift your mindset and focus on self-improvement.

Positive affirmations or mantras can be a powerful tool to shift your mindset and focus on self-improvement after getting out of a negative relationship instead of constantly checking on your ex. Firstly, positive affirmations help to rewire your thought patterns and beliefs. By consciously repeating positive statements about yourself and your capabilities, you can challenge and replace any negative or self-limiting thoughts that may have resulted from the toxic relationship. This practice helps boost self-esteem, foster self-belief, and cultivate a positive mindset essential for personal growth and healing.

Secondly, positive affirmations constantly remind you of your worth and value. They help you to reconnect with your strengths, resilience, and inner qualities that may have been overshadowed in the toxic relationship. By affirming your worth and focusing on your positive attributes, you reinforce a sense of self-love and self-acceptance. This shift in mindset enables you to let go of the past and embrace a future filled with self-improvement, personal growth, and new possibilities.

Lastly, using positive affirmations or mantras creates a proactive and empowering mindset. It encourages you to take charge of your thoughts and emotions and actively engage in self-improvement. By repeating positive statements about yourself and your desired outcomes, you set clear intentions and create a roadmap for personal development. This practice helps to foster resilience, motivation, and a sense of empowerment as you navigate the journey of healing and moving forward.

In summary, incorporating positive affirmations or mantras into your daily routine can be transformative after getting out of a negative relationship. It helps to rewire your thought patterns, reconnect with your worth, and cultivate a proactive and empowering mindset. By using positive statements about yourself and your potential, you shift your focus towards self-improvement, personal growth, and a brighter future. This practice empowers you to let go of the past, embrace self-love, and create a positive narrative that supports your healing and transformation.

12 Steps to Recovering from A Toxic Relationship

Set healthy boundaries with your ex and communicate clearly about your needs and expectations.

Setting healthy boundaries with your ex and communicating your needs and expectations is crucial after getting out of a negative relationship instead of constantly checking on them. Firstly, setting boundaries protects your emotional well-being and promotes your personal growth. It allows you to create a safe space for yourself and establish limits on acceptable and respectful behavior. By clearly communicating your boundaries to your ex, you establish a foundation of self-respect and assertiveness, essential for moving forward healthily and positively.

Secondly, setting boundaries helps to maintain your independence and autonomy. It allows you to prioritize your needs and focus on your personal development without getting entangled in the dynamics of the past relationship. By clearly expressing your expectations and limits, you create a space to freely explore your path and make decisions that align with your values and goals. This empowers you to reclaim your sense of self and rebuild your life on your terms.

Lastly, setting boundaries with your ex promotes healing and closure. It allows you to detach emotionally and create space for healing. By clearly communicating your needs and expectations, you set the stage for productive and respectful interactions, reducing the chances of getting caught up in toxic patterns or unresolved issues. This enables you to move forward and find closure as you establish new boundaries that support your well-being and reflect your growth after the toxic relationship.

In summary, setting healthy boundaries with your ex and communicating clearly about your needs and expectations is essential after leaving a negative relationship. It protects your emotional well-being, promotes personal growth and independence, and facilitates healing and closure. By setting boundaries, you create a safe space for yourself, prioritize your needs, and assert your autonomy. This empowers you to move forward healthily and positively, free from the negative dynamics of the past relationship, and with a renewed focus on your well-being and personal development.

Focus on personal growth and development, such as taking a class or pursuing a new career opportunity.

Focusing on personal growth and development, such as taking a class or pursuing a new career opportunity, is a powerful way to shift your focus away from checking on your ex and toward your self-improvement. Firstly, investing in personal growth allows you to redirect your energy toward positive and productive endeavors. By engaging in activities that expand your knowledge, skills, and experiences, you open doors to new opportunities and possibilities. This boosts your self-confidence and helps you discover new passions and interests that can bring fulfillment and joy into your life.

12 Steps to Recovering from A Toxic Relationship

Secondly, focusing on personal growth and development promotes self-discovery and self-empowerment. It encourages you to explore your talents, strengths, and values and align your life with what truly matters to you. Investing in yourself creates a sense of purpose and direction, which can be immensely liberating and empowering. Instead of dwelling on the past or seeking validation from your ex, you take charge of your life and create a future aligned with your authentic self.

Lastly, focusing on personal growth allows you to build a strong foundation for your future. Investing in your education, skills, and career enhances your prospects for success and fulfillment. Whether taking a class to acquire new knowledge, pursuing certification to enhance your professional skills, or exploring a new career opportunity, each step toward personal growth opens new doors for advancement and personal satisfaction. This improves your self-worth and builds resilience and confidence, enabling you to easily navigate future challenges.

In conclusion, focusing on personal growth and development after getting out of a negative relationship is a transformative and empowering choice. It allows you to channel your energy towards positive and productive endeavors, discover your true passions and values, and build a strong foundation for your future. Investing in yourself and embracing growth opportunities creates a pathway to self-empowerment and personal fulfillment. Instead of checking on your ex and dwelling on the past, you redirect your focus toward creating a brighter, more rewarding future for yourself.

Ending a toxic relationship can be difficult and emotional, and the urge to check in on an ex-partner can be overwhelming. However, there are several ways to resist this urge and protect your emotional well-being. One effective strategy is to remove your ex's contact information and unfollow them on social media. This can reduce the temptation to check in and limit exposure to triggers that may bring up painful memories or emotions. It can also help establish healthy boundaries and create personal growth and healing space.

Another helpful strategy is to focus on your own self-care and emotional well-being. This can include engaging in positive self-talk, seeking professional help, journaling, and practicing mindfulness or meditation. By taking care of yourself and prioritizing your needs, you can build resilience and inner strength and cultivate a sense of self-worth and confidence that is not dependent on your ex. Ultimately, the key to resisting the urge to check in on your ex after a toxic breakup is to prioritize your healing and growth and to establish healthy boundaries that protect your emotional well-being and allow you to move forward with positivity and hope.

12 Steps to Recovering from A Toxic Relationship

"Don't Check On Your Ex Quotes"

"You can spend minutes, hours, days, weeks, or even months over-analyzing a situation, trying to put the pieces together, justifying what could've, would've happened... or you can just leave the pieces on the floor and move the f*** on."— **Tupac Shakur.**

Additional Resources - I

Here are some resources for additional support for people in or getting out of toxic relationships:

Therapy options:

Private Sessions with Keith K. L. Belvin: Free Discovery Session Form: *https://bit.ly/KeithBelvinProfessionalLinks* Take a few moments to answer all the questions. Your answers will allow Mr. Belvin to understand what is happening in your life. In addition, by answering all the questions in detail, Mr. Belvin will learn what to offer in your current time of need.

Psychology Today: *https://www.psychologytoday.com* This website has a directory of therapists where you can search for someone who specializes in helping people dealing with toxic relationships.

BetterHelp: *https://www.betterhelp.com* This online therapy platform provides affordable and accessible therapy services. They have licensed therapists who specialize in various areas, including relationships.

National Domestic Violence Hotline: *1-800-799-7233* The hotline provides support and resources for people experiencing domestic abuse or violence. In addition, they can connect you to local resources, including counseling services.

12 Steps to Recovering from A Toxic Relationship

Online communities:

r/AbuseInterrupted:
https://www.reddit.com/r/AbuseInterrupted
This subreddit community provides support, resources, and education for people dealing with abuse in their relationships.

Love is Respect: *https://www.loveisrespect.org.* This website offers a safe and anonymous online chat service for people experiencing relationship abuse. They also have a blog section that covers a wide range of relationship topics, including healthy relationships, red flags, and communication.

One Love Foundation: *https://www.joinonelove.org* The site educates young people about healthy and unhealthy relationships. In addition, they have an online community where you can connect with others going through similar experiences.

Recommended reading:

"Our Bond Is Our Gift" by Keith K. L. Belvin, MHSC, MS Ed.

Based on popular Periscope and Facebook live videos, Our Bond Is Our Gift is a book for those men and women ready to roll up their sleeves and dig in and do the work to become good men and women for themselves, their relationships, their families, and their communities.

Additional Resources - I

Here are some resources for additional support for people in or getting out of toxic relationships:

Therapy options:

Private Sessions with Keith K. L. Belvin: Free Discovery Session Form: *https://bit.ly/KeithBelvinProfessionalLinks* Take a few moments to answer all the questions. Your answers will allow Mr. Belvin to understand what is happening in your life. In addition, by answering all the questions in detail, Mr. Belvin will learn what to offer in your current time of need.

Psychology Today: *https://www.psychologytoday.com* This website has a directory of therapists where you can search for someone who specializes in helping people dealing with toxic relationships.

BetterHelp: *https://www.betterhelp.com* This online therapy platform provides affordable and accessible therapy services. They have licensed therapists who specialize in various areas, including relationships.

National Domestic Violence Hotline: *1-800-799-7233* The hotline provides support and resources for people experiencing domestic abuse or violence. In addition, they can connect you to local resources, including counseling services.

12 Steps to Recovering from A Toxic Relationship

Online communities:

r/AbuseInterrupted:
https://www.reddit.com/r/AbuseInterrupted
This subreddit community provides support, resources, and education for people dealing with abuse in their relationships.

Love is Respect: *https://www.loveisrespect.org.* This website offers a safe and anonymous online chat service for people experiencing relationship abuse. They also have a blog section that covers a wide range of relationship topics, including healthy relationships, red flags, and communication.

One Love Foundation: *https://www.joinonelove.org* The site educates young people about healthy and unhealthy relationships. In addition, they have an online community where you can connect with others going through similar experiences.

Recommended reading:

"Our Bond Is Our Gift" by Keith K. L. Belvin, MHSC, MS Ed.

Based on popular Periscope and Facebook live videos, Our Bond Is Our Gift is a book for those men and women ready to roll up their sleeves and dig in and do the work to become good men and women for themselves, their relationships, their families, and their communities.

"Why Does He Do That?" by Lundy Bancroft: This book offers insight into the mindset and tactics of abusive men. It also provides practical advice for those trying to leave an abusive relationship.

"The Verbally Abusive Relationship" by Patricia Evans:
This book focuses on the insidious nature of verbal abuse and provides strategies for dealing with it.

"Healing from Hidden Abuse" by Shannon Thomas: This book explores the impact of emotional abuse on victims and guides how to heal and move forward. It's important to remember that leaving a toxic relationship can be difficult and may require professional support. Call emergency services if you or someone you know is in immediate danger.

Additional Resources - II.

Here is a guide outlining common traits of toxic partners to help you recognize red flags in future relationships:

Here Are The Red Flags:

Lack of Empathy:

Toxic partners often lack empathy. They don't understand or care about your feelings and may dismiss or make fun of them. They may also be unable to see things from your perspective.

Controlling Behavior:

A toxic partner may try to control what you do, whom you see, and where you go. They may be possessive and jealous, trying to isolate you from your friends and family.

Verbal Abuse:

Verbal abuse is a common trait of a toxic partner. They may belittle you, insult you, or call you names. They may also gaslight you, making you doubt your sanity or memory.

Manipulative Behavior:

A toxic partner may manipulate you to get what they want. They may use guilt, shame, or other emotional tactics to control you. They may also try to make you feel responsible for their happiness or well-being.

Lack of Respect:

A toxic partner may disrespect you in various ways. They may be rude, dismissive, or condescending towards you. They may also disregard your opinions or feelings.

Inconsistent Behavior:

A toxic partner may have erratic behavior, mood swings, or emotional instability. They may be affectionate one moment and distant the next, making it difficult for you to understand what they want or need.

Narcissistic Traits:

A toxic partner may have narcissistic traits, such as being self-centered, having a sense of entitlement, and lacking empathy. They may also be obsessed with their appearance, status, or achievements.

Blaming and Criticizing:

A toxic partner may blame you for their problems or criticize you excessively. They may refuse to take responsibility for their actions and make you feel guilty for things that are not your fault.

Isolating Behavior:

A toxic partner may try to isolate you from your friends, family, or hobbies. They may discourage you from pursuing your interests or spending time with people who care about you.

12 Steps to Recovering from A Toxic Relationship

Physical Abuse:

Physical abuse is a severe and dangerous trait of a toxic partner. It can include hitting, slapping, pushing, or other violence. If you experience physical abuse, it's crucial to seek help immediately.

Recognizing these red flags can help you avoid toxic partners and build healthier relationships. Remember, identifying the negative signs and seeking support and help to get out safely is essential in a toxic relationship.

Keith L. Belvin

Who Is Keith K. L. Belvin, MHSC, MS Ed.?

Keith's Bio

Keith K. L. Belvin is a certified Crisis Specialist, Personal & Marriage Counselor, Award-Winning Author, and Educational Consultant who listens to and helps address emotional problems through Person-Centered Counseling. Keith collaborates with men, women, children, and couples by addressing their current issues and works to help them become experts in their lives and feelings. In addition, Keith helps mentor many to become more self-aware of how powerful they are and was created to be. Keith's friendly and transparent style makes him the perfect person to open up to and communicate your problem.

If you require Professional Counseling, don't hesitate to reach out and set up a Free Discovery Counseling Call with Keith K. L. Belvin; go to the following link:

https://bit.ly/KeithBelvinProfessionalLinks

Websites & Emails:

Counseling and Consultant Info:

www.BravinConsultants.com

Counseling Email: **info@BravinConsultants.com**

Books, Publishing, & Literary Services:

12 Steps to Recovering from A Toxic Relationship

www.BravinPublishing.com

Publishing Email:

MainOffice@BravinPublishing.com

Professional and Personal Highlights:

Owner of Bravin Consultants LLC and Bravin Publishing

www.BravinConsultants.com & www.BravinPublishing.com

Crisis Specialist, Professional Counselor, Certified Marriage Counselor, Professional Problem Solver

Weekly Live Show on Tik Tok, Fridays, 11:30 am - 1:30 pm **https://www.tiktok.com/@keithklBelvin**

Creator, Owner, and Director of The **Young Kings & Queens After-School Mentor Program**. A traveling program designed to help correct harmful behaviors and the choices connected to them.

Award-Winning Published Author. (available at www.Bravinpublishing.com)

Frequent Literary Contributor to multiple anthologies, including The Soul of a Man series (2009 Anthology of the Year Award). Keith is also featured in volumes #2 & 3 in The Soul of Man. Word Play 1: Words are our Canvas—international poetry anthology contest winner 2013. (available at www.Bravinpublishing.com or anywhere books are sold)

Keith L. Belvin

Contracted by the Bureau of Alcohol, Tobacco, Firearms and Explosives, provided workshops and direct counseling for field officers and employees in need of assistance.

Keith is an award-winning poet featured in the US and Europe.

Masters in human service counseling, specializing in Christian Ministry, Liberty U.

Masters in education, Walden U

Former Dean of Students & Educator, NYCDOE, 1995 to 2016

Featured in Ebony Magazine's Black Love issue 2012.

Signed to Black Expression Book Club and featured in Ebony, Jet, and Essence magazines. 2011

Certified Educator Delaware & New York

Certified Investigator for the State of Delaware

Happily, Married Man of God. Twenty-three years, married to my wife, Tiffany, and father of seven children, ranging from 40 to 9 years old. As discussed in detail in his book "From Gigolo to Jesus."

Keith's Social Media Links.

Tic Tok:

https://www.tiktok.com/@keithklbelvin

YouTube:

https://www.youtube.com/c/KlBelvin

Facebook:

https://www.facebook.com/KeithKLBelvin/

Instagram:

https://www.instagram.com/keithklbelvin/

Clubhouse:

https://www.clubhouse.com/@keithklbelvin

Twitter

https://twitter.com/KeithKLBelvin

LinkedIn

https://www.linkedin.com/in/keithbelvin/

Keith L. Belvin

Keith K. L. Belvin's Literary Titles & Merch

Keith K. L. Belvin's Titles Can Be Purchased on his websites, and anywhere books are sold worldwide.

www.BravinConsultants.com - **Counseling & Consultants Services**

www.BravinPublishing.com - **Publishing Services**

www.amazon.com/shops/TheBravinConsultantsstore - **Amazon Store**

Here are Keith's other titles for you to add to your library:

A Man in Transition by K. L. – *Poetry (Keith's first published book in 2008, Award Winning Poems)*

From Gigolo to Jesus, From Misogyny to Monogamy – *Memoir*

Lukewarm Saint 1 – *Inspirational Fiction*

Our Bond Is Our Gift - *Relationship Self Help*

The Choice – *Romantic Short*

Future Titles Coming Soon:

From Gigolo to Jesus, 10 Steps to Personal Growth and Spiritual Transformation – *Self Help*

Lukewarm Saint 2: Fox in The Hen House – *Inspirational Fiction*

You, Me, Us, - Making Marriage – *Marital Support*

12 Steps to Recovering from A Toxic Relationship

Anthology Contributions:

The Soul of a Man (Book #1) – *Inspirational Collaboration (2009 award winner, Best Anthology of the Year)*

The Soul of Man (#2) – *Inspirational Collaboration (Runner of 2015 Best Anthology of the Year award)*

The Soul of Man (#3) – *Inspirational Collaboration (2021)*

Word Play 1: Words Are Our Canvas – *Poetic Collaboration*

Word Play 2: The Foundation of *Soul* – *Poetic Collaboration*

No Test No Testimony: In Times Like These: A Look Back at *2020* - *Reflective Collaboration*

Being A Black Man, It's Harder than You Think: Inspirational Collaboration (2023 award winner) – *Inspirational Collaboration*

Bravin Apparel:

Clothing and Accessories

 - https://bit.ly/BravinApparel

"Don't suffer in silence. Together We Can Fix This, If You Bring Me Your Pain."

Keith K. L. Belvin, MHSC, MS Ed.

#WeCanFixThis